LET'S GET PHYSICAL
Puzzle No. 35

```
O  L  K  E  C  S  P  U  H  S  U  P  G  F  Q
C  T  O  N  I  N  G  D  R  K  G  S  I  Y  C
A  Z  U  M  B  A  H  B  A  N  P  T  E  S  M
R  P  A  O  G  D  A  C  I  N  N  Y  X  W  T
D  S  S  O  K  R  L  G  T  E  C  K  E  I  S
I  E  Y  C  B  R  G  L  S  E  A  E  R  M  L
O  T  P  E  I  O  O  S  I  R  R  R  C  M  R
Q  A  L  P  J  B  O  W  A  M  O  T  I  I  U
B  L  R  O  L  E  O  T  A  R  D  S  S  N  C
S  I  R  R  A  Q  E  R  H  K  U  A  E  G  G
F  P  K  P  S  I  N  N  E  T  J  V  E  U  E
I  H  C  I  A  T  X  S  T  A  U  Q  S  R  L
Y  E  I  K  N  R  E  N  I  A  R  T  M  I  T
C  U  D  S  F  G  E  S  R  S  P  U  T  I  S
```

AEROBICS	BARBELLS	BIKING	CARDIO
DANCE	EXERCISE	FITNESS	GYM
JOGGING	JUDO	KARATE	LEG CURLS
LEOTARDS	PILATES	PUSHUPS	SITUPS
SKIP ROPE	SQUATS	STRETCH	SWIMMING
TAI CHI	TENNIS	TONING	TRAINER
TREADMILL	WORKOUT	YOGA	ZUMBA

CORN...
Puzzle No. 36

```
M E F W T Z M I S K E R N E L
D L E I Y O K V C G X P T Y M
H W E S O Y R E D W O H C E N
C A B R E U G T K V L D A K D
R L B B O K R R I A O L G S O
A H C L O E A L E L N F N I K
T H F B M C E L S L L S I H F
S K O O G D E R F H L A D W S
N B V L A Y E H X K E A D Z N
A E D L E T M Q T S S P U S I
R R A C T G I M A N T U P T F
Z S E I H S I L E R O I H C F
S Y R U P N S M R I H Y R X U
K F B T C A S S E R O L E G M
```

ALLERGY	BEEF	BREAD	BROOM
CASSEROLE	CHOWDER	DOGS	FLAKES
FLOUR	FRITTERS	GRITS	HOLE
HUSK	KERNEL	MEAL	MUFFINS
ON THE COB	PUDDING	RELISH	REMOVER
SALAD	SALSA	SNAKE	STARCH
SYRUP	TORTILLA	WHISKEY	YIELD

DOWN MAIN STREET

Puzzle No. 37

```
Y  L  C  I  L  B  U  P  O  H  U  M  Z  F  K
A  G  S  C  A  O  R  F  M  L  U  K  W  E  I
D  S  N  W  O  L  C  O  L  S  G  F  S  S  U
I  T  P  I  S  S  C  J  I  A  I  S  T  T  D
L  I  R  D  H  C  T  C  U  R  G  A  R  I  Q
O  E  N  A  A  C  C  U  E  B  O  S  E  V  S
H  A  C  S  D  H  R  T  M  L  I  D  E  A  N
B  C  I  I  E  I  R  A  F  E  A  L  T  L  O
Q  O  X  E  L  U  T  L  M  R  S  H  E  E  O
N  R  R  X  C  O  A  I  A  N  D  O  O  E  L
U  S  O  K  O  P  P  P  O  F  B  R  Q  H  L
S  D  W  O  R  C  Z  F  N  N  R  S  U  B  A
W  J  E  S  U  A  L  P  P  A  D  E  R  M  B
R  A  L  U  P  O  P  I  I  H  Z  S  R  T  S
```

APPLAUSE	BALLOONS	BANDS	CHEERS
CLOWNS	COSTUMES	CROWDS	DRUMS
FESTIVAL	FIRE TRUCK	FLAGS	FLOATS
HOLIDAY	HORSES	JUBILEE	MARCHING
MUSIC	OCCASION	PARADE	POLICE
POPULAR	PUBLIC	STREET	TRADITION

G-WHIZ!
Puzzle No. 38

```
J  G  S  B  N  G  U  G  E  A  E  C  A  R  G
L  L  B  S  O  U  U  S  N  G  R  G  M  I  A
G  A  L  L  O  N  O  E  I  L  N  A  M  B  B
E  D  F  Q  K  O  T  F  L  S  E  L  E  H  A
B  E  G  E  G  A  N  A  O  G  D  A  O  G  R
R  B  E  U  U  I  B  Y  U  J  L  X  G  X  D
V  R  E  D  A  M  Z  A  S  L  O  Y  H  Y  I
G  G  A  N  U  R  C  M  B  P  G  D  O  T  N
R  R  R  G  O  A  D  J  O  A  Y  G  S  E  E
G  R  J  O  M  T  A  O  G  Z  R  G  T  G  C
N  V  G  O  W  T  S  A  N  M  Y  G  J  D  O
A  D  L  L  D  P  M  M  E  J  W  X  J  A  Q
T  E  Y  M  U  E  H  F  E  T  N  A  I  G  Q
P  G  R  U  T  E  L  B  I  G  P  N  S  R  C
```

GABARDINE	GADGET	GALAXY	GALLON
GAME	GEAR	GEMSTONE	GHOST
GIANT	GIBLET	GIZMO	GLAD
GLUE	GNAT	GOAT	GOLDEN
GOLFER	GOOSE	GRAB	GRACE
GRADUATE	GREEK	GROW	GUACAMOLE
GUARD	GUMBALL	GYMNAST	GYPSY

ANNIVERSARY PARTY

Puzzle No. 39

```
S E T A D L M N G N I L R A D
J D I C Y E N O H C U K M H M
E L N M J Z F I I F A U A J Y
W F L O W E R S S E U R L G D
E O E O B B S S C K M I D F N
L H G T Q S I A T O F S Y S A
R A A D X L R P N E D S P E C
Y P I X B B H Y L E D E C S C
P P R Z M N E O V E C N R S L
R I R E R S N O V B A D A I U
O N A N U G T O Y M H N H K F
M E M O Z I L X O S Y I U Z Y
U S P T O E J R P O T K G T O
H S G N B E T A R B E L E C J
```

BELOVED	BLISSFUL	BONDS	CANDY
CARDS	CELEBRATE	DARLING	DATE
DEVOTION	EMBRACE	FLOWERS	HAPPINESS
HARMONY	HONEY	HUMOR	JEWELRY
JOYFUL	KINDNESS	KISSES	LIFELONG
MARRIAGE	PASSION	ROMANCE	SPOUSE

WIZARD OF OZ
Puzzle No. 40

```
S Y E K N O M A G N I Y L F B
M F T F D R E A M W C T N R W
Q R R J C Z D E O N I U A S S
Y Q A E Y N Z O R E S I M R A
H R E F I B D W I L N U N E S
T A H L S S U O I C I N I P N
O I G S M H O R Y Y K C T P A
R N X A C O D C R C H L F I K
O B N T N U A E M I C E Q L X
D O I D U S N R L B N H O S M
E W Y E M E R A L D U E T O B
M E G A R U O C Z G M N O I L
Y P E E L S T S N U L R T V X
N M E E I T N U A D B Y M W Z
```

AUNTIE EM	BICYCLE	BRAIN	BROOM
COURAGE	DOROTHY	DREAM	EMERALD
FARM	FLYING	GLINDA	HEART
HOUSE	KANSAS	LION	MONKEYS
MUNCHKINS	RAINBOW	RUBY	SCARECROW
SLEEPY	SLIPPERS	TIN MAN	TORNADO
TOTO	UNCLE HENRY	WITCH	WOODSMAN

SEND IN THE CLOWNS

Puzzle No. 41

```
A O C K N K R C N R O C P O P
U N T E K C I T T S V A B S X
D S E P U R N I E T L C N I J
I B Z R C R G V D N P R J D L
E A E U A H M C R U T O E E K
N T S A T U A P A T R B L S N
C R H R R N S G T S S A C H I
E A O A N S T B O R Y T Y O A
J P Z O A P E M E T A S C W T
E E N J O N R L L X R B I Z R
M Z C T O Q G W F N I O N F E
S E G A K G S R E G I T U Y T
H I H U U G O D N R O C F P N
B U C J M U N R A B S T A G E
```

ACROBATS	ARENA	AUDIENCE	BARNUM
BEARS	BIG TOP	CANNON	CIRCUS
CORN DOG	ENTERTAIN	JUGGLERS	LEOTARD
POPCORN	RINGMASTER	SIDESHOW	STAGE
STUNTS	TENT	TICKET	TIGERS
TIGHTROPE	TRAPEZE	TROUPE	UNICYCLE

WHAT'S IN "CHOCOLATE PIE"?

Puzzle No. 42

```
M  J  O  L  O  C  C  I  P  Q  E  H  O  P  E
T  J  O  B  E  N  M  V  O  N  M  P  A  L  O
U  P  C  J  L  E  P  A  H  C  H  T  A  A  T
R  P  A  C  E  C  I  M  S  R  I  N  P  C  L
J  Z  T  N  O  E  C  I  L  O  P  L  K  E  A
E  L  O  C  H  I  L  A  T  C  H  C  A  P  C
M  T  O  T  O  T  P  O  U  F  H  I  M  C  I
E  A  A  H  O  O  O  H  W  O  T  L  P  D  T
W  P  C  L  E  H  P  L  T  T  S  O  L  B  P
B  E  J  S  P  A  P  E  C  S  T  H  O  E  O
C  A  P  I  T  O  L  L  F  H  G  T  L  P  C
T  C  T  X  E  F  A  L  O  C  F  A  A  X  E
P  H  N  L  P  P  C  L  R  U  T  C  H  M  Q
G  A  O  A  L  O  E  D  N  Q  H  C  A  O  C
```

ALOE	CALICO	CAPE	CAPITOL
CATHOLIC	CHAPEL	CLOTH	COACH
COCOA	COLA	ECHO	HALO
HOPE	HOTEL	ICECAP	LACE
LATCH	OLEO	OPAL	OPTICAL
PATIO	PEACH	PHOTO	PICCOLO
PLATE	POLICE	POTHOLE	TACO

Contents

Recipes

INTRODUCTION

I was first diagnosed with gout at the young tender age of 26 years old and boy was my first attack was painful and crippling. When my doctor first diagnosed me, I refused to believe it was gout, thinking to myself that I must get a second opinion, that it must be a fracture of some type. Why would a 26 year old get gout at such an early age? Yes at the time I was overweight by about 40 pounds and I loved to indulge at McDonalds or some other grease joint. I also loved to drink! Jack Daniels whisky with Coke was my choice of beverage at the bars on the weekends and yes, I was young and when you are young, you think that you are immortal, death seems far away but the truth is, we aren't... and my diagnosis of gout was the real wake-up call that things had to change in my life.

Funny thing is, all of my gout attacks have been correlated with me drinking JDs and Coke few hours before each and every attack! My lifestyle desperately needed to change, I remember after another bout with a gout attack going to visit another doctor and jokingly telling my girlfriend at the time that I was "expired, finished!" "Time to get rid of this guy and find somebody else", he laughingly said. I was shocked to hear those comments although he was a bit rude in my opinion but you know what? He said the truth! Some people don't like to hear the truth, I know cause I've told friends who are overweight that if you continue in your ways you will have health issues but they simply disregard me. It's like listening to a doomsdayer calling for the end-times in their ears! They kind of look at you like you are nuts! There is so much confusion out there about what is considered good to eat and bad to eat, so many diets that contradict each other and so much bad advice in the media, on the internet, magazines sometimes even from your own doctor.

So I set up to learn, learn and learn some more and test, test and test some more to see what works and what doesn't, I've spoken to countless doctors over the years and in this e-book you will find my findings basically on how to live with your gout and lower those uric acid levels to avoid another gout attack. Now I know what you are thinking? You're thinking: "Tell us about how to cure gout and how get rid of this disease". Truth be told, not all of yous, who are gout sufferers can cure gout. For example, if you have a blood disorder like *thalassemia* or *anemia*, you will most likely never get rid of your gout and should never attempt to try and cure your gout through diet. Truth be told that is the reason I got gout at such an early age was due to the fact that I was born with *thalassemia minor* and I am just a tad anemic due to the thalassemia. Studies have shown that people who have a blood condition are more prone to develop gout later in life so for me unfortunately it's a genetic thing, whereby I can't reverse my gout through an extreme dietary change, it's like fighting a losing battle, there is no point, I am too sensitive. Plain and simple.

A stern warning for those who are on prescription drugs like allopurinol, colchicine, probenecid and want to get off of them through remedies and/or dietary change. **By doing so you will most likely get a gout attack or several gout attacks as your body adjusts getting off of the medication**.You can try it but the method I suggest is the following:

Step 1
Talk to your doctor about it beforehand and see if he is willing to work with you in monitoring your progress. If he has good reason not to since you may have another condition then listen to him and do not attempt to get off your meds. The recommended way is to lower your prescription drug doses progressively, measuring the results of your blood tests. Anything that is done abruptly will backfire with a gout attack!

Step 2
If you find your doctor is simply ignorant to the recommendation then try and find another doctor who is willing to monitor your progress and give it a try.

Step 3
Regular blood tests will need to be done on a regular basis to monitor any progress.

Step 4
Follow all the dietary information in this e-book and stick to the diet. This also means no smoking and no drinking alcohol whatsoever.

Step 5
Drink nothing else but water, one cup of coffee or tea a day is allowed.

<u>Step 6</u>

Exercise, do whatever you enjoy, just make sure to exercise.

<u>Step 7</u>

If you think you've beaten gout, then write to me, I'd like to hear your story, I might even interview you sometime for a future post on my website. You can contact me at info@goutandyou.com

I can't stress it enough! I have tried and failed. **Remember the more gout attacks you get, chances are you can eventually damage your joints permanently.** Furthermore, don't think that by taking allopurinol that you are out of the woods. The unseen side effects include increases of overall acidity in the body, which puts extra burden on your kidneys, liver and other organs. Think every time you take your allopurinol, you are slowly poisoning your body, eventually you will have to pay the price by risking kidney or liver failure. There is risk involved for sure but I was never a fan of not taking risks and simply doing what one told you to do and leaving it at that. Why? Cause **I believe in the body's ability to heal!** There are so many examples of people that have been healed from their condition whether it's diabetes, high blood pressure, gout, cardiovascular disease and yes even cancer! I've spoken to so many doctors and other health professionals who have witnessed drastic turnarounds in health through the body's ability to heal through proper diet and exercise. But truth be told, not all will succeed due to the fact that our bodies are all different, the conditions we may have varies from one and another, pre-existing conditions come into play like genetics, your environment also plays a role, my version of gout and your version can be totally different as well as the progression of the disease inside our bodies.

So what's the point of me reading this book you say? Plenty! My uric acid levels went from sky-high where I was taking 300mg of the prescription drug allopurinol and 2mg a day of the other prescription drug colchicine to **only taking 100mg of allopurinol daily!** Not bad for a guy with a blood disorder and now my uric acid levels have stabilised! For the first time in my life I am in control of my disease and battle with gout and you can be too if you follow the information on the lifestyle change I have compiled for you. Make no mistake about it, there is no cure-all remedy for gout. In the long term it won't fly! Maybe in the short term you can get some relief but in the long term it's coming back. Your uric acid levels will only respond if you change your lifestyle and nothing else.

What do you mean by lifestyle Spiro? I mean look at yourself in the mirror and don't lie to yourself. If you are overweight you gotta begin dropping the pounds. If you smoke it is time to butt out! If you are stressed it is time to rid of the problem causing you the stress. Check out my post on stress. If you love to drink it is time to limit your alcohol intake, if you want to avoid those painful gout attacks. If you have a sweet tooth for things all sugar, best you limit that or face other diseases other than gout down the road.

This e-book will teach you the right way to eat and live a healthier, happier life. Most importantly I will dispel some common myths about food that the masses get wrong. I'll give you an example. I always advocated that we consume no more than 5% of our calories as sugar, say about 25mg a day max. Obviously, some people barked at such an assumption since no medical authority has come out publicly to state such an opinion yet. Well as of March 5th 2014, the World Health Organization came out with a new recommendation that sugar should be no more than 5% of your daily calories and since 2002 they've been recommending 10% of your daily calories can be sugar. Truth is most people consume more than 10% of their daily calories in sugar and that is tragic. Many of these people will go on to develop gout, diabetes and other diseases if they don't change their ways.

Remember in the 1970s how the government fought the battle against fat saying it was the main culprit in fighting diseases like cancer and food companies started removing fat from foods that naturally had them like cheese, milk, yogurt and even butter recommending it being replaced with margarine. I remember my mom buying margarine in the 1980s, everybody was buying it and look at the destruction it's done to the health of so many people. Now medical authorities have changed their mind again by keeping the fat that naturally occurs in cheese, milk and yogurt and labelling it as a healthy food to eat again, hence the greek yogurt craze! This type of meddling creates the ball of confusion we live in today.

Nowadays, poor gluten is taking the beating! The market for gluten-free products is exploding and we don't know exactly why. Many people perceive gluten-free as simply healthier but that is far from the truth. In fact a gluten-free diet isn't healthier! If you have celiac disease which 1% of Americans do, the condition which is caused by an abnormal immune response to gluten then I would say yes, eat gluten-free! But for the rest of us, by eating gluten-free we are essentially taking out the vitamins, minerals and fiber from wheat which is the most important part!!! This is the stupidity that I am going to straighten out for you in this e-book, I know it's a dirty job but somebody has to do it. What I fear the most is that we have lost our common sense about what is good to eat and what simply isn't. I will make this e-book very simple for you to understand, even a 6 year old can understand what a good diet should consist of regardless if you suffer from gout, diabetes, hypertension, cardiovascular disease etc...

What this e-book will cover is the major diseases that are killing our people today like coronary heart disease, diabetes, high blood pressure, osteoporosis and even cancer. Why you ask? Because people with these diseases end up developing gout later on or vice versa. There are many gout sufferers who are diabetic, suffer from hypertension, have issues with their heart or developed gout after suffering from osteoporosis. There are also dietary instructions for those who suffer from those diseases as well. We will also put fat, protein and carbohydrates under the microscope and analyze them properly. We need to get the story straight and stop the confusion. Enough bullshit! You will get the correct information on how to feed your body and what to feed your body on a daily basis in order to live with lower uric acid levels, to limit gout attacks and other potential diseases, that can develop from the bad eating habits you developed. The e-book will also touch upon smoking, alcohol and exercise, as well as the corruption of Big Pharma and those greedy food companies.

The goal of this e-book is not to cure you from gout but to lower your uric acid levels and stabilise them on the lower end of the spectrum, in conjunction with your doctor's urate lowering therapy. This will put less stress on your joints, you will be able to live without any gout attacks and will lead you to living a healthier life overall. If you follow these dietary instructions, you will also avoid any risk of developing other diseases like diabetes, high blood pressure, heart disease, stroke and osteoporosis which are all linked with gout. For those who read my posts on the blog, I don't want to repeat the same topics, home remedies and other tips that you can find there, so you won't find much here. This is more of a detailed explanation of my post titled "Gout diet" that goes a long way providing you all the juicy details about eating right and living healthier, happier and much smarter.

What is Gout?

Historically, gout was referred as "the king of diseases and the disease of kings" or "rich man's disease" and its' first documentation goes back all the way to 2600 BC Egypt. Why? It's obvious that royalty and the rich could afford meats, alcohol and liked to fatten themselves up with other rich foods, as for the lower class they were stuck with a carbohydrate diet, whatever fruits and vegetables they raised on their land, rarely eating any meat but living a healthier life! Several hundred years ago, gout was also thought to be caused by drops of viscous humors that seeped from blood into the joints. The word Gout is derived from Latin word gutta meaning "a drop of liquid" and has the unique distinction of being one of the most frequently recorded medical illnesses throughout history. A good article I read recently in HistoryToday.com provides a great summary:

Gout, the 18th century's signature condition, is on the rise in contemporary Britain, with a 60 per cent increase in the last 15 years. In the Georgian era gout's association with luxurious living led to its status as a badge of honour or a signal the sufferer had reached a certain level in society. As the physician William Heberden commented: 'This seems to be the favourite disease of the present age in England, wished for by those who have it not, and boasted of by those who fancy they have it.' In contrast, today's manifestation of the disease is associated with the nutritional effects of poverty rather than affluence.

Undoubtedly a painful condition, gout usually begins with acute pain and swelling in the big toe and then extends to other joints such as fingers, often accompanied by feverish sweating. Eighteenth-century cartoons of corpulent gentlemen with their feet in buckets or up on footstools may look comical, but the truth is that the ailment is excruciating and disabling. Richard Grenville wrote in a letter to his sister Hester Pitt (whose husband also suffered the complaint): 'Gout is gone but has left me such a swelling quite up to the top of my Thigh, as does not seem even disposed to abate.' Three weeks later: 'I can walk almost without a stick, but have still a swell'd Leg, the remains of gout; a swelld hand and lame arm which keep me confined.' Sufferers were predominantly male, although older women were also susceptible, so we find Sarah Churchill writing towards the end of her life: 'I would desire no more pleasure than to walk about my gardens and parks; but, alas! that is not permitted; for I am generally wrapped up in flannel, and wheeled up and down my rooms in a chair. I cannot be very solicitous for life upon such terms, when I can only live to have more fits of the gout.'

Nevertheless, on some occasions gout was actively desired, as the belief was that it was incompatible with and would therefore drive out other illnesses. Horace Walpole called it 'a remedy and not a disease'. Betsy Sheridan, sister of the playwright Richard Brinsley Sheridan, wrote to her sister Alicia LeFanu: 'My Father is at last thank God fairly in the Gout – And has received the congratulations of Dr Millman on the occasion. The fact is that all his Phisicians have wish'd for this event but seem'd fearfull that he had not strength enough to throw off his disorders in that way.'

Gout had many disguises. Roy Porter and G.S. Rousseau identified over 60 different types in one 18th-century treatise, including 'galloping gouts' and 'flying gouts'. Other conditions were falsely labelled gout, including headaches and stomach complaints; the belief was that it came about as the result of an excess of one of the four humours flowing (or 'dropping', since the name is derived from the Latin gutta, a drop) to a weakened area of the body. Consequently gout was considered to be caused by 'a sedentary life, drinking too freely of tartarous wines; irregular living, excess in venery; and obstructed perspiration and a supression of the natural evacuations'. Now we know that gout results from too much uric acid in the blood, either because an excess is produced or the kidneys are not filtering it efficiently. It can be worsened by the consumption of foods rich in purines, including anchovies, venison and goose – all of which featured strongly in the 18th-century diet of the better off. Then, as now, obesity and a high alcohol intake are contributory factors.

William Rowley's provocative treatise The Gout Alleviated (1770) compares 'a gentleman of fortune' – who feasts on 'wild fowl, made dishes, rich sauces, puddings, tarts, &c. with glasses of various liquors' – with 'a poor man', who during a hard day's work contents himself with 'meat, if it be attainable ... a little strong or small beer' and bread and cheese for supper. It is thus almost natural, in Rowley's view, that: 'The generality of men of fashion have the gout before they are 50 ... The gout is scarce ever seen amongst the lower order of people.' Today the greatest number of gout cases are found in the north-east of England, an area with the highest level of unemployment and of alcohol-related illness.

Modern drugs to treat gout include the anti-inflammatory Colchicine, which has as its active ingredient the poisonous extract of autumn crocus, from the same genus as the hermodactyl that was used for this purpose by the ancient Greeks. Some 17th-century recipes for curing gout do include hermodactyl, but by the 1700s it was discarded as potentially dangerous until Nicolas Husson, an officer in the French army, concocted a quack remedy called Eau Medicinale, which had colchicum as one of its secret ingredients and was adopted enthusiastically by the medical establishment around 1820. Instead, the 18th-century remedies mainly focus on soothing the inflammation through poultices and purges. A Dr Cook's 'recipe for the gout' dating from 1769 was simply a blend of onion juice and vinegar, heated and applied to the area of pain. Dr Clark of Edinburgh's remedy of eating two or three red herrings before going to bed and his instruction to chew straw for the accompanying violent thirst would have been likely to make the problem worse. More palatable might be Margaretta Bampfylde's suggestion of tea made from speedwell buds, which 'if you make it too strong it will have the same effect as an opiate'.

There was also a stress on the right diet, something that sufferers are advised to consider today. A Dutch physician, Herman Boerhaave, prescribed milk and bread or porridge for breakfast and supper, with only barley, oats, rice or millet and vegetables for dinner, not too dissimilar to the current NHS recommendations. It would certainly have been more successful than the 'regimen to prevent the gout' followed by Sir Edward Filmer, who restricted himself to eating 'what ever was most agreeable to his appetite' capped by '4 or 5 glasses of good strong red port wine'.

What causes gout exactly?

What causes gout is excess uric acid in the body and is one of the most painful form of arthritis. It's a complex disorder that is more prevalent among men, and afflicts women more commonly after menopause. Besides men have higher uric acid levels in their blood than women, that's why nearly 6% of men have it and 2% of women in the US. That's about 8 million Americans that have gout! Gout is a kind of arthritis caused by a buildup of uric acid crystals in the joints. Uric acid has no useful function in the human body; it is simply a breakdown product of purines, a group of chemicals present in all body tissues and many foods. Uric acid is a breakdown product of purines that are part of many foods we eat mostly found in meats, seafood etc... An abnormality in handling uric acid and crystallization of these compounds in joints can cause attacks of painful arthritis, kidney stones, and blockage of the kidney filtering tubules with uric acid crystals and can lead to eventual kidney failure. Most of the time uric acid dissolves and goes into the urine via the kidneys. However, if the body is producing too much uric acid, or if the kidneys are not excreting enough uric acid, it builds up. The accumulation results in sharp urate crystals which look like needles.(1) They accumulate in the joints or surrounding tissue and cause pain, inflammation and swelling. They accumulate in the joints or surrounding tissue and cause pain, inflammation and swelling. It's usually characterized by recurrent attacks of acute inflammatory arthritis—a red, tender, hot, swollen joint (God knows I've had many) and the most commonly affected area is the big toe 50% of the time and is called podagra. Other joints that can be affected include the ankles, knees, wrists, fingers, heels and elbows and it is wise to always rest the joint that hurts as much as possible. In some people, the acute pain is so intense that even a bed sheet on the toe causes severe pain. I've personally have had sleepless nights of tossing and turning, trying to numb the pain with a bag of ice. Usually, the gout attacks occur in the middle of the night, supposedly the coolness and temperature drop facilitates the crystallization of the uric acid in the joint.

Digging deeper, high levels of uric acid in the blood called Hyperuricemia is the underlying cause of gout. Surprisingly, hyperuricemia is commonly found in many people who never develop gout. Scientists are not completely sure what causes hyperuricemia. There is definitely a genetic factor because a person who has close relatives with hyperuricemia is more likely to develop it himself or you had the same bad eating habits as your dad or mom and developed it that way.

To confirm a diagnosis of gout, your doctor may draw a sample of fluid from an inflamed joint to look for crystals associated with gout or do a blood test to measure the amount of uric acid in the blood.

Who's at risk?

Finally, you are more likely to have gout if you are a male, obese, is in your family genes, drink excessive alcohol, eat foods high in purines, regular aspirin, niacin or diuretics use, hypertension, lead poisoning, surgery etc... Complications can also arise from gout like recurrent gout, advanced gout in which urate crystals may form under the skin in nodules otherwise known as tophi, kidney stones may cause urate crystals to accumulate in the urinary tract, gout may also spread to other joints and obviously cause damage to the joints.

The 4 Stages of Gout

Medical professionals have broken down the development of gout in four stages, how the disease can evolve over time. First stage is what they call Asymptomatic Gout the stage where somebody develops hyperuricemia which is higher uric acid levels in the blood, the body becomes increasingly acidic but no symptoms are present. At this stage, uric acid crystallizes and silently accumulates in the joint. Treatment is not required at this stage and no medication is required but if you do find out by taking a blood test, that you do suffer from hyperuricemia, a change in your diet should take place immediately.

Second stage is the very first gout attack. What they call Acute Gout or Acute Gouty Arthritis. Yes your first time comes to a shock and is excruciatingly painful causing severe inflammation and severe pain in the joint. Before that night where you got your gout attack, you consumed something like seafood, organ meat, had too many Cokes or a night of drinking that raised your uric acid levels which triggered your gout attack. Even stress or the presence of another illness can cause it too! The pain will escalate over the next 8 to 12 hours making walking very difficult. Generally, this gout attack will be in the big toe area and will feel like a broken foot. The inflamed area will be reddish and you can experience a slight fever or even chills. You should find some relief after three days but symptoms can hang around up to 10 days and sometimes even longer. These attacks can then become more severe and prolonged if nothing is done about them. The next acute attack can take months or more than a year to reoccur. Over time, however, attacks can last longer and occur more frequently.

Next up is the third stage, what they call Intercritical Gout or Interval Gout which is the period of time in between gout attacks where you feel no symptoms and your joints function properly. Life is great and you feel great but everything is just an illusion! For most gout sufferers, uric acid in the blood remains high and the crystals remain in the joint. The truth is gout hasn't gone away and the low levels of inflammation between attacks may be causing you joint damage even if you do not feel any symptoms or pain. In addition, a low level of inflammation could be associated with the risk of developing heart disease or even a stroke! These delayed attacks can be far more threatening than the initial attack and will move to different joint areas such as the Achilles area. It is essential to seek proper medical treatment for the disease and change your lifestyle through proper diet and exercise to avoid and/or prevent any future gout attacks.

Finally, we end it with the final and fourth stage, what they call Chronic Gout or Chronic Tophaceous Gout which is the stage you definitely want to avoid at all costs. At this stage gout becomes disabling and occurs after many years of suffering that can be associated with irreversible damage to the affected joints, damage to your kidneys and even death! Over time gout attacks become longer and more frequent. This is the worst and most destructive stage due to the fact that you can develop tophi causing the destruction of the affected bone and cartilage to occur. This stage usually occurs after 10 years if the disease hasn't been treated properly and no lifestyle changes were implemented. With proper treatment most gout sufferers do not progress to this stage and thank goodness for that! It is critical that you treat gout in the earlier stages.

Chapter 1:

Fat, Protein & Carbs...Getting the

Facts Straight

Ok, let's get started here and dig in a simple controversy a few years back about oat bran. A study came out which basically stated that oat bran is so good for you. It was added in cereals, and there was a lot of rave about it. Then another study came out stating that oat bran is no better than anything else. It is the soluble and insoluble fiber that occurs in most of the fruits and vegetables that are good. Now whether it's oat which is mostly a soluble fiber, or wheat which is mostly an insoluble fiber, it doesn't really matter because our body needs to enjoy a variety of foods. If mother nature created it for us, then it is good for us. Let's not just overdo things and be a glutton about it, because too much of anything, at the end is no good.

To read more about the fiber content of different foods, check out this link: http://huhs.harvard.edu/assets/file/ourservices/service_nutrition_fiber.pdf

Our body is a masterpiece creation with excess capacity. The human brain contains about 10 billion nerve cells or neurons, each capable of storing 40 billion memories. We lose a few couple hundred daily depending how we abuse our brain from food and drink. Our body also has two kidneys and we can live with only one of them functioning, if we have to. We also have two lungs which enable us to breathe in oxygen which is very important for metabolism. Our body has excess capacity for all of our vital organs and yet we abuse them so badly that sometimes we wear them out in only 30 to 60 years!!! We all know of a love one or friend that has passed away way too soon and way too young. This is the greatest tragedy any person can experience!

Fat and blood from meats are concentrates that the body cannot tolerate in great quantities. In digesting them, we produce so many waste products that even our kidneys which have excess capacity cannot handle them properly and that results in diseases. Excess fat is your number one health enemy!

Exercise profits us by making us feel better, relaxing us and pushing our bodies to live longer.So lesson number two is that, lack of exercise is your second health enemy. Get up and exercise, it energizes your body! Go out for a walk instead of lying in front of the boob tube. Take the stairs instead of the elevator, join the gym, participate in sports and you will be much healthier and feel so much better. But most importantly, do an activity you enjoy and do it with others. Make your activity a social event, it is so important to connect with other human beings for your mental health also! So get up and exercise you will feel energized!

Next up many of yous have gotten gout from eating those organ meats. My message to you is very simple, no fatty organs for you, period. So what's wrong with these organs? We have discovered that it stores as it detoxifies the food we eat. Detoxification is something our bodies do on a daily basis. It is the process of eliminating toxins through the five eliminatory channels: liver, colon, lungs, kidneys, lymph and skin. Eating organ meats increases your uric acid levels. Cut them off!

In the world we live in today, with polluted water, air and food, our bodies regularly get overloaded with substances that are harmful to it –they are called toxins! As our bodies become overloaded, they are also overburdened with eliminating these toxins so that many undesirable substances stay in our bodies.

Surrounding these invading substances with mucous and fat is one way our system tries to shield us from there harmful effects. A good portion of these harmful substances are stored in our fat deposits! There is an exception to the function of fats, our body has over 40 billion fat cells in it and they help cushion the vital organs and insulate us from the cold. Cholesterol is an important molecule in the body, but did you know that most of the cholesterol needed by our bodies is made by our own liver? The remaining cholesterol is obtained through the foods we consume, it comes from the fruits and vegetables that we eat and our body manufactures it in the liver.

Even if we don't take in any cholesterol at all and take in those fats that do not have cholesterol in them, unfortunately our body manufactures it! So it's easy to get too much. Persistently high cholesterol levels can be detrimental to our heart and blood vessels. Various poisons from insecticides and fertilizers that are used in agricultural products become concentrated in the liver as well as the kidneys, so that it takes seven times as much water for the kidneys to detoxify fats and proteins as it does for carbohydrates.

What are carbohydrates after all? Too many people have confused it with calories. For example, they say potatoes don't have as many calories as an apple. I say, with food that has grown from the earth, you can eat as much as you desire because it's good for you.

What about animal meat? The animal consumes food from the earth and then processes it in its' own body, and gives us a concentrate of fat. As a general rule, you have to avoid concentrates of all forms and <u>fat is a concentrate</u>. You have to remember that excess fats are our number one health enemy; so if you want to be healthy avoid it altogether. Eighty percent of all the major illnesses and diseases today can be prevented. We can cut the death rate now if we change our intake with the proper food. What should we eat then?

Clean meat in principle, has nothing bad in it and you can continue to eat it. The unclean animals that are mother nature's scavengers and part of their role is garbage collection and as such, we shouldn't take them in our bodies otherwise, we partake of their unclean nature. What are some of those unclean meats? Number one on the list is swine, pig, hog, bacon, ham and pork.

Check out what Wikipedia has to say on the subject: (http://en.wikipedia.org/wiki/Pigs)

"Pigs can harbour a range of parasites and diseases that can be transmitted to humans. These include trichinosis, Taenia solium, cysticercosis, and brucellosis. Pigs are also known to host large concentrations of parasitic ascarid worms in their digestive tract. The presence of these diseases and parasites is one reason pork meat should always be well cooked or cured before eating. Today, trichinellosis infections from eating pork are relatively uncommon, at least in the United States, due to more stringent health laws, better refrigeration, and public awareness of the dangers of eating undercooked meat. Some religious groups that consider pork unclean refer to these issues as support for their views. Pigs are susceptible to bronchitis and pneumonia. They have small lungs in relation

to their body size; for this reason, bronchitis or pneumonia can kill a pig quickly.[19] There is concern that pigs may allow animal viruses such as influenza or Ebola to infect humans more easily. Some strains of influenza are endemic in pigs (see swine influenza), and pigs also can acquire human influenza."

Do I have your attention now? Other unclean meats are the squirrel, the turtle, mouse, rat and frog which are becoming fashionable in certain parts of the world to eat nowadays from what I'm reading in the papers, especially in Asia.. When it comes to fish we need to eat fish that lack fangs and have scales, fish that do not meet this criteria are fish like the catfish, shark, piranha, sturgeon, crab and lobster, shrimp, oysters, scallops, birds of prey like the buzzard, hawk, swan and woodpecker. What is it that they cause you ask; well very simply: sickness, illness and disease. These are animals that eat other dead animals and other garbage. It's no wonder that lobster was once considered the cockroach of the ocean and now it's considered as the best supposed quality fish meat. Yet if you eat lobster, crab, shrimp, oysters...your blood uric acid levels will rise. Why? It's not considered healthy food for your body. Plain and simple.

What are examples of clean meat? Beef, lamb, deer, goat and fish that don't have fangs but have scales that are clean, bass, blue fish, cod, haddock, halibut, herring, mackerel, snapper, trout, salmon, perch, sole and chickens with their eggs, birds like quail and turkey, just to name a few. It is not needful that we can eat all of those; the point is that there are many clean meats that you can choose from. Never diet, meaning to starve yourself but eat safe proper food, don't go hungry, don't skip meals but enjoy every bite.

Avoid concentrates such as sugar and fat. Fat is a concentration of various poisons. As animal store fats, they also store along with it many of the poisons that we have scattered in the environment. It concentrates everything that is not good for us including cholesterol.

You often see in advertisements from food companies who claim that the oils they use are cholesterol-free. But what they didn't tell you is that the oil they use is actually 100% fat, and that, is definitely not good for you. Remember that the food industry is dollar driven and because of that you can expect deception all of the time. They will tell you lies in such a manner that you will believe it because it's mixed with half-truths. For example, they say: "This food is cholesterol free." Cholesterol only occurs in animal products. None of the vegetable oils have cholesterol in them but since they are all fats, it's bad for you in spite of what the American Heart Association tells you, stating that 30% of calories coming from fat is fine. But the truth of the matter is, only 10% of fat is ideal, because that's all that the body can cope with!

If you have a disease like cancer, you'll have to strive for the ideal. Meaning, that you should have no visible fat in your body, and as a rule of thumb, you should stick with below 2 grams of fat per serving. Processed foods have too much fat in them. You can eat as many of the naturally grown foods as you possibly can, but you need to permanently cut off on all the fats if you happen to have any disease.

Enjoy complex carbohydrates that the earth has given us like fruits, vegetables and grains. Don't go hungry but rather enjoy food! There's over 100 delicious recipes for you to enjoy in this e-book. Fill yourself up! Eliminate the fat; it has more than twice as many calories per gram compared to carbohydrates and protein combined. Let's take a slice of whole wheat bread for comparison and yes, it's good for you. It has 70 calories per slice, eat as much as you like, it has only 1 gram of fat, 3 grams of protein and 16 grams of carbohydrates. Carbs is pure energy; it burns clean and has very few waste products. Only carbon dioxide and water are cleaner! It's passed out of your urine, sweat, breathing, perspiring while working. You breathe out carbon dioxide, so it doesn't stress the vital organs like the liver and kidneys and so on. Meat generally has 70-75% of its calories as fats, eggs 70-75% also, cheese has about 70%, fruits only 3%, vegetables about 5%, grains about 5% also, rice 4% and oatmeal 15%.

Vegetable oils are all 100% fat, therefore, they are very bad for you. I repeat very bad for emphasis sake. It is true that animal fats have cholesterol in them; all animal products have it like meat, eggs, butter, milk, cheese etc. Does that mean we shouldn't use any of them? Of course not! If we are sick, we should cut on them drastically. If we don't want to get sick, we should cut back on them mildly. Animal fats also cause coronary heart/artery disease and vegetable fats cause cancer. As much as seven times more cases of cancer are caused by this and then further developed by animal fats. Let's take olive oil as an example, it's a monounsaturated fat and has the good cholesterol called HDL and has very little LDL. If you want to have good cholesterol levels, you have to go out and exercise. Have a sweet tooth? Heat up some oatmeal and add a teaspoon of raw honey in it and don't feel guilty about it. Raw Honey has only 15 calories per teaspoon and has many nutrients in it, but try to avoid sugar as much as you can. You can also add sliced bananas, raisins and pitted prunes, even a couple of teaspoons of concentrated apple juice to sweeten it. Always sweeten it wisely. Oat bran, bran in all grains and cereals that's made from whole grains is good for us.

You'll never get everything 100% right, none of us do; we all fail from time to time. So don't feel guilty if you eat some wrong foods or over indulge at a wedding reception, at a party or at home. But try to stay focused on enjoying great health as much as you can because this involves self-discipline on your end. Keep trying, some folks I know and myself included, took a few years to stay on a healthy food eating plan based on mostly carbs, so don't give up. Our body gets tempted from time to time to eat what we know is not good for us, but tastes so darn good!

The ideal gout diet should consist of the following formula: **Eighty percent of your calories should be carbohydrates, the energy food!!! Ten percent of your calories should be fat and the remaining 10% should be protein.**

It takes more water to separate the waste products from the protein but your principal food should be carbs like veggies, fruits, grains, whole grain breads, beans, corn, whole wheat pasta and rice. Anything you can grow in your garden is good for you and you can eat all that you want from it. Stop listening to the mainstream media and what this expert and that expert says, they are all confused anyway!

Now going back to vegetable oils, let's look at a good example. At the other end of olive oil, let's take corn oil for example. It is a concentrate. It takes 14 ears of corn to make one tablespoon of vegetable oil and then we heat it under intense heat that it changes the oil, this is not good for you beloved. If you add 2-3 tablespoons of corn oil in something that you are cooking, you are in trouble beloved.

So how then can we cook our foods? If you have an egg, you are better off boiling it at a temperature of 212 degrees F. If you fry them by adding grease, you increase the free radicals which cause diseases. The same thing is true if you scramble them and that's why, always eat your eggs soft boiled.

How should we eat meat? Ideally, cook your meat over fire with a BBQ, all the fat will be gone with the smoke and that's how you get rid of the cholesterol. The manner in which your meat is cooked also counts in the cholesterol department. Frying your meat is probably the worst way to prepare meat if you are trying to follow a low-fat diet. Meats that are fried are also high in saturated fat, which can increase your cholesterol levels. Instead, try baking, broiling, or roasting your meat. These methods can also deliver some tasty dishes and will not sabotage your cholesterol-lowering efforts as badly as frying your meat.

What about fish? Fish is the best source of protein and has very little fat. It averages from 3-5% fats and the rest of its' calories are proteins. They say that diseases are hereditary. But they are not hereditary at all, rather, we have inherited the bad habits of choosing improper foods and we have developed diseases as we processed them. Am I saying that we should eat our food unprocessed or uncooked? No, but if you stick to fresh food from the garden, fruits and vegetables, frozen foods, canned fruits and so on, you'll feel healthy and live healthy.

Now let's learn to calculate the percentage of fat in marketing ads and on labels. Remember to always calculate on weight and not percentage. For example, milk chocolate has 54% of calories coming from fats, but you need to calculate for one piece, 2 pieces or the entire chocolate bar. Expect deception from advertising and the food companies. There is talk now from the federal government to change the present system of food labelling.

How to Calculate Percentage of Calories from Fat, Carbohydrates and Protein

Step 1
Obtain the amount of fat, carbohydrates and protein in a serving of the food. The nutritional label should provide these values in units of grams.

Step 2
Derive the number of calories in the food that come from fat. Each gram of fat provides about 9 calories, so the number of calories that come from fat is 9 x F, where F is the number of grams of fat. Assume the food has 11 g of fat. The food, therefore, provides 9 x 11 = 99 calories from fat.

Step 3

Compute the number of calories that come from carbohydrates. Each gram of carbohydrates provides about 4 calories, so the number of calories that comes from carbohydrates is 4 x C, where C is the number of grams of carbohydrates. Assume the food has 7 g of carbohydrates. The food, therefore, provides 4 x 7 = 28 calories from carbohydrates.

Step 4

Compute the number of calories that come from protein. Each gram of protein provides about 4 calories, so the number of calories that come from protein is 4 x P, where P is the number of grams of protein. Assume the food has 8 g of protein. The food, therefore, provides 4 x 8 = 32 calories from protein.

Step 5

Find the total number of calories in the food. This will be the sum of the calories from fat, carbohydrates and protein. A food that has 99 calories from fat, 28 calories from carbohydrates and 32 calories from protein will have a total of 99 + 28 + 32 = 159 calories.

Chapter 2:

CORONARY HEART DISEASE—The

Number One Human Killer & Its' Link

With Gout

Your body has roughly 60,000 miles of blood vessels and when they start becoming clogged, they gradually close off. As a vessel closes, blood goes into it more rapidly, kind of like sludge that developed on the wall of the artery. A typical American male of 25 years of age has already closed 25% of his coronary artery lumen. We eat as much as 40-50% of our calories as fat and where it should have been around 10%. Trim all the fat from the meat, cook your food properly, broiled away and don't overheat it as you cook it. "Well done" will be sufficient in order to remove all the blood. Oxygen capacity is lesser when the arteries are clogged risking also a stroke. When you reduce fat in your diet, you will notice your immune system gains more and more strength. So eat no fat and make sure you eat lean meats. The fats that are the worst are the animal fats that have cholesterol in them like meat, butter, cheese and milk. Cholesterol is the principal cause of coronary heart disease and it kills roughly 600,000 people in the US every year—that's 1 in every 4 deaths. More than half of the deaths due to heart disease in 2009 were in men. Coronary heart disease is the most common type of heart disease, killing more than 385,000 people annually. Every year about 935,000 Americans have a heart attack. Of these, 610,000 are a first heart attack. 325,000 happen in people who have already had a heart attack according to the United States Centers for Disease Control and Prevention. Sadly, many of them suffered from gout too! Coronary heart disease is not a hereditary disease but a result of bad eating habits, avoid the confusion that is out there.

When you pass out after you have eaten too much, this is due to eating too much fat. Not enough oxygen is getting into the brain; again I reiterate to eat more carbohydrates in your diet. What about polyunsaturated fats such as margarine, corn oil, Crisco, sunflower oil, coconut oil, palm oil, peanut oil and many others? Although they don't cause coronary heart disease that badly, they do cause other diseases like cancer. Just Google the keywords "polyunsaturated fat and cancer" to see the many studies that consistently show a link between polyunsaturated fats to higher cancer risks. Don't take my word for it, check it out for yourself!

The American Heart Association and the American Diabetes Association will tell you to switch from animal fats to vegetable fats to avoid coronary heart disease. This is completely wrong! Leave both the animal fats and vegetable fats since they both cause diseases like different types of cancer. While you decrease your risk of coronary heart disease you also increase your risk of cancer. There's as high as seven times more cancer deaths from those who eat polyunsaturated fats compared to those who eat animal fats. While it's true that we decrease coronary heart disease by about 10%, but this is not the right way. What you need to do is to cut your fat intake to 10% of your daily caloric allowance because this will lower your blood cholesterol within 3 weeks and you will decrease the risk of heart attack by 50%. Doctors can decrease them with medicines and diet so that in 3 years, you will have only reduced the risk by 5% to 10%. What do you want, the truth or the consequences?

Prevention is the key! If we know how to prevent this disease, we are better off than trying to treat it after we already have it. This is not taking away from your doctor, it is very important to monitor your health condition but he won't be able cure you. That responsibility is yours, although there are some very knowledgeable doctors who know the true facts but they are rare. Remember they got forced-fed in college to learn a certain way and not criticize the establishment of PhDs who wrote their textbooks, so their ignorance is obvious. Also, look at your personal doctor. Does he look like somebody who watches his health, is your doctor obese, smoke, drink or takes prescription drugs himself to treat a disease? If yes, you need to find another doctor, someone who practices what they preach.

The simple road to health is to eat a very low fat diet, exercise regularly and to stop smoking. Know that smokers are about seven times as apt to develop coronary heart disease than non-smokers. Going back to carbs, they have barely any fat, they are pure energy, there are very few waste products and our metabolism burns them clean. They don't lay plaques in your arteries like fat so make them 80% of your daily caloric intake. Yes I am repeating myself but I want to make sure that you engrave the message of this e-book in your brain.

Now the North American diet is about status; eating big burgers, big steaks and hot dog contests wherein a person can eat as many Wieners in a setting as he can. This is the trend for the past few years; supersize your fries, supersize your cola etc. The number one source of fat in the American diet is meat, second is milk, third is cheese and fourth is vegetable oil. Each percent of your total cholesterol that goes down, your risk of coronary heart disease goes down by 2%. So in just 3 weeks on a proper food diet, you can reduce your blood cholesterol by 25%. Does this mean you should monitor your cholesterol every week? Of course not! If we reduce the fatty foods we ingest which primarily comes from animal fats, our cholesterol will go down. Ideal cholesterol is "100" plus your age and in no case over "150". If it doesn't go over "200" you are doing rather well. I urge to check out some of the town studies that were done over many decades in Framingham, Massachusetts. One particular study states that if your cholesterol is "200" or less there is not much risk in developing these diseases, if it goes over "200", your risk goes up rapidly, "213" your risk goes up fivefold, "230" your risk goes up 6.7 times and clocking in at "255", your risk is 12 times as great! Twelve people die out of every "100" that had cholesterol over "250". Fifteen out of every "100" people die every year if their cholesterol count was "300"! People with cholesterol level over "260" have 4 times the risk of coronary heart disease than those who have "200". Without medicine, you can reduce your total cholesterol level by 25% in 3 weeks with proper diet and your risk drops by 50% (check out their website at www.framinghamheartstudy.org for a wealth of information). The key to prevention is proper food and not medicine, not money and not your doctor.

Fiber is the hero! Both soluble and insoluble fibers are indigestible. They are therefore not absorbed into the bloodstream. Instead of being used for energy, fiber is excreted from our bodies. Soluble fiber forms a gel when mixed with liquid, while insoluble fiber does not. Insoluble fiber passes through our intestines largely intact. It is good for the stool and speeds up the flow through your bowel by cutting the time it transits the bowel from about 90 hours to about 33 hours. It also allows you less time to absorb things like fat and cholesterol, so it's very helpful. Wheat has insoluble fibers as well as vegetables such as green beans and dark green leafy vegetables, fruit skins and root vegetable skins, whole-wheat products, wheat bran, corn bran, seeds and nuts. Soluble fibers come from oat/oat bran, dried beans and peas, nuts, barley, flax seed, fruits such as oranges and apples, vegetables such as carrots and psyllium husk. They mix with the cholesterol and allow you to absorb less of it as you eat more and more soluble fiber. Magnesium does the same; it occurs in hard water wells and prevents the absorption of fat and cholesterol. It unites with cholesterol and causes it to pass through your stool, moving its bulk through the intestines, controlling and balancing the pH (acidity) levels in the intestines. Here's a deeper study on magnesium from www.magnesiumforlife.com:

"If you're ever rushed to the hospital with a heart attack, intravenous magnesium could save your life. In a 1995 study, researchers found that the in-hospital death rate of those receiving IV magnesium was one-fourth that of those who received standard treatment alone. In 2003, a follow-up study of these same patients revealed an enduring effect of magnesium treatment. Nearly twice as many patients in the standard treatment group had died compared to those who received magnesium, and there were considerably more cases of heart failure and impaired heart function in the placebo group. In addition to increasing survival after heart attack, IV magnesium smoothes out arrhythmias and improves outcomes in patients undergoing angioplasty with stent placement.

Magnesium is absolutely essential for the proper functioning of the heart. Magnesium's role in preventing heart disease and strokes is generally well accepted, yet cardiologists have not gotten up to speed with its use. Magnesium was first shown to be of value in the treatment of cardiac arrhythmias in 1935. Since then there have been numerous double-blind studies showing that magnesium is beneficial for many types of arrhythmias 23 including atrial fibrillation, ventricular premature contractions, ventricular tachycardia, and severe ventricular arrhythmias. Magnesium supplementation is also helpful in angina due to either a spasm of the coronary artery or atherosclerosis.

Heart palpitations, "flutters" or racing heart, otherwise called arrhythmias, usually clear up quite dramatically on 500 milligrams of magnesium citrate (or aspartate) once or twice daily or faster if given intravenously.- Dr. H. Ray Evers

A magnesium deficiency is closely associated with cardiovascular disease. Lower magnesium concentrations have been found in heart attack patients and administration of magnesium has proven beneficial in treating ventricular arrhythmias. Fatal heart attacks are more common in areas where the water supply is deficient in magnesium and the average intake through the diet is often significantly less than the 200-400 milligrams required daily. Magnesium is proving to be very important in the maintenance of heart health and in the treatment of heart disease. Magnesium, calcium, and potassium are all effective in lowering blood pressure. Magnesium is useful in preventing death from heart attack and protects against further heart attacks. It also reduces the frequency and severity of ventricular arrhythmias and helps prevent complications after bypass surgery. Magnesium deficiency appears to have caused eight million sudden coronary deaths in America during the period 1940-1994. - Paul Mason Researchers from Northwestern University School of Medicine in Chicago have determined that not having enough magnesium in your diet increases your chances of developing coronary artery disease. In a study of 2,977 men and women, researchers used ultrafast computed tomography (CT scans) of the chest to assess the participants' coronary artery calcium levels. Measurements were taken at the start of the study—when the participants were 18- to 30-years old—and again 15 years later. The study concluded that dietary magnesium intake was inversely related to coronary artery calcium levels. Coronary artery calcium is considered an indicator of the blocked-artery disease known as atherosclerosis.

Almost all adults are concerned about the condition of their heart and cardiovascular system. Some live in constant fear wondering whether any ache, cramp or pain in their upper body is a sign of a heart attack. There isn't an adult living in North America that hasn't lost a loved one or a family member to heart disease. The fact is heart attacks kill millions every year.

Chernow et al in a study of postoperative ICU patients found that the death rate was reduced from 41% to 13% for patients without hypomagnesemia (low magnesium levels). Other post heart surgery studies showed that patients with hypomagnesemia experienced more rhythm disorders. Time on the ventilator was longer, and morbidity was higher than for patients with normal magnesium levels. Another study showed that a greater than 10% reduction of serum and intracellular magnesium concentrations was associated with a higher rate of postoperative ventricular arrhythmias. The administration of magnesium decreases the frequency of postoperative rhythm disorders after cardiac surgery. Magnesium has proven its value as an adjuvant in postoperative analgesia. Patients receiving Mg required less morphine, had less discomfort and slept better during the first 48 hours than those receiving morphine alone.

It is established that clinically significant changes in a number of electrolytes occur in patients with congestive heart failure (CHF). Magnesium ions are an essential requirement for many enzyme systems, and clearly magnesium deficiency is a major risk factor for survival of CHF patients. In animal experiments, magnesium has been shown to be involved in several steps of the atherosclerotic process, and magnesium ions play an extremely important role in CHF and various cardiac arrhythmias.

Magnesium is also required for muscle relaxation.Lower magnesium levels can result in symptoms ranging from tachycardia and fibrillation to constriction of the arteries, angina, and instant death. Due to lack of magnesium the heart muscle can develop a spasm or cramp and stops beating. Most people, including doctors, don't know it, but without sufficient magnesium we will die. It is important to understand that our life span will be seriously reduced if we run without sufficient magnesium in our cells and one of the principle ways our lives are cut short is through cardiac arrest (heart attack). Yet when someone dies of a heart attack doctors never say "He died from Magnesium Deficiency." Allopathic medicine ignores the true causes of death and disease and in the field of cardiology this is telling. Magnesium is an important protective factor for death from acute myocardial infarction."

Source from www.magnesiumforlife.com (check website for indexation)

So to summarize, eat both soluble and insoluble fibers and some magnesium from time to time. Eat in moderation every food that has fat in it. Our brain is made of 100% cholesterol; another exception is children under the age of 2 years old because they need fats to develop their brains and tissue. What about pasta? Pasta, rice, oatmeal, cream of wheat is all good for you. Make sure to eat plenty of fish which has plenty of protein and cold pressed olive oil.

Olive oil lowers blood pressure and blood cholesterol, it raises the HDL or good cholesterol, does the opposite of other oils and reduces our blood sugar, so naturally it is good for diabetics, gout sufferers and it prevents heart disease. Substitute olive oil for other oils in your baking and salad dressings; add it over pasta or a baked potato because it is the only exception to fats. If heated, it loses its healthy benefits and produces free radicals that cause us to develop diseases like cancer. Look at the fast food industry when we fry in the same grease all day long, over and over. Maybe it is polyunsaturated oil but if you heat it, it will cause you problems. Avoid all kinds of fats; nuts consists of 75% of its calories as fat, fish about 3-5%, butter 99%, whole milk 45%, 2% milk only has 30% of its calories as fat, skim milk only 2%, ice cream usually around 85%. Don't believe the frozen yogurt deception that says it has no fat because in checking, you will find that 22% of its calories consist of fat. Beef and lamb has about 70%, skinned chicken is only at 15% because it is white meat. Trim the fat off from the beef and try to eat more free range beef instead of corned beef because cows that eat grass is always a better choice. Run or walk for 3 miles a day at least 3 to 5 times a week. That's about a 45 minute walk.

Chapter 3:

Preventing Cancer - What You

Should Know As a Gout Sufferer

People and medical professionals are confused and research goes out into all directions but with little to no results. Think of all of the money we donate to different charities, foundations and hospitals who are looking to develop the latest medication in order to cure us of our sicknesses.

A study from exercise physiologist Doug Paddon-Jones from the University of Texas Medical Branch concluded that from an Ironman triathlon competition, eating 4 ounces of meat a day was adequate to rebuild the muscles that athletes would wear out during training. The need for more protein is exaggerated particularly in advertisements and many athletes believed that more protein is better. When we eat too much protein, its' metabolism produces ammonia, urea and other waste products, that take seven to eight times more water to flush out through the kidneys than carbohydrates. Consuming too much meat is also a culprit in gout. Truth is you don't need too much protein in your diet, 4 ounces of meat is more than enough, so as a gout sufferer make you sure you cut it down and eat more fresh carbohydrates.

Animal products are the only ones that have cholesterol in them and are the number one factor in the development of coronary heart disease. The big mistake is to replace animal fat with polyunsaturated fat like vegetable oil that will help reduce coronary heart disease but increases the risk of cancer. It will reduce the risk of coronary heart disease by 5-10%, but on the other hand, the risk of cancer then goes up to 50-70%— you are decreasing one disease and increasing another. Beware of processed foods that use vegetable oil because as they subject the oil to high temperature, they destroy its value. Stop eating those fried chicken nuggets, French fries, white rice (replace it with basmati or wild rice instead), potato chips, deli meats. Also, as a very strong concentrate, fat has 2 ½ times as many calories per gram compared to carbohydrates and protein.

On the other hand, when you eat carbohydrates, your body metabolizes 20% of it as energy and stores the rest as fat. Even if you overindulge in carbohydrates, it is very difficult for the body to store it as fat. But if you eat fat on the other hand, it's very simple and little conversion is needed. Remember that fat is your number one health enemy and number two is lack of exercise. Coronary heart disease is caused by ingested fat which hardens in the arteries. Most of the degenerative diseases are caused by the digestion of dietary fats like coronary heart disease, cancer, diabetes, high blood pressure and atherosclerosis. They result in the depletion of oxygen to the vital organs and we begin to get sick because we are not getting the proper nutrients. **Eighty percent of these diseases including gout can be prevented right now!** With proper diet and adequate exercise with no smoking, we can eliminate 80% of these illnesses that plague us right now! Can you believe that? If you remove those bad foods from your diet, you will immediately begin to get relief as quickly as 72 hours, with marked improvement noticed in the efficiency in which you carry oxygen in the vital organs. It is your responsibility to take out all the visible fat from your diet. The world simply is drowning in information but is starved for wisdom, knowledge and understanding of the true facts. Do not expect good health to come to you in capsules! Real meaningful prevention is ignored; nutrition is the major factor in such things as health and disease. Somehow the medical profession doesn't want to accept that your body is truly your best doctor and that nutrition is the major factor in disease prevention and that in reality, we are what we eat and our immune system will really work if we avoid the fat. Listen to it! Look how a fracture heals itself without any problem, the body heals itself and heals fast.

Animal fats and saturated fats are basically a solid at room temperature while polyunsaturated fats are liquid and then we hydrogenate them to make them solids for our margarines and oleo. Of course that takes additional heating and creates additional problems for our health. Why is butter a lot better than margarine? It is because of the heating process that we subject margarine to—into a manufacturing process that gets to such high temperatures—that the free radicals increase and cause more disease. Prevention is the key! Butter is an exception to the rule if we eat it in moderate quantities because of the fact that it has not been processed. Why is that you ask? The cow doesn't overheat it; she never gets it to more than her body temperature. What is buttermilk, anyway? Originally it was simply the liquid left over after whole milk or cream had been churned into butter. The churn's motion caused the butterfat to separate from the milk or cream which solidifies into butter. The liquid that remained is called buttermilk. So butter is ok for us to eat and it provides us with the good type of cholesterol called HDL, which allows the building of brain tissues, fibers that cover the nerve sheaths and all the cell membranes that cover them. Nutrition is the super factor and the cornerstone of prevention. Nutrition is the answer to cancer as well as gout. It's the foods you eat! Cancer kills 21% and heart disease kills 52% every year; that is a total of 73% of all deaths caused by these 2 main diseases. Many of these people who have died from these 2 diseases have also suffered from gout. When you develop gout, consider it as a strong warning signal that if you continue your bad eating habits that you too, are headed towards the road of bad health and even death! You now have an opportunity to educate yourself and follow a healthy gout diet plan, include some exercise and lower those deadly uric acid levels that can destroy you.

Eighty percent of diseases are preventable with no drugs, no money and no doctor visits but just by avoiding fat. So read the labels on foods carefully and watch for the number of grams of fats per serving. By eliminating fat from your diet, you will eliminate 50% of cancers with this step alone while you will eliminate 30% of it if you stop smoking. Cancers caused by fat are colon cancer, cancer of the uterus, breast cancer, ovarian cancer, prostate cancer and pancreatic cancer—all caused primarily by dietary fats. As we metabolize fat, bile salts are produced. While it is true that bile salts are necessary to digest the fat, but they are also carcinogenic and proved to cause colon cancer.

What do we eat then? We eat a diet that is high in soluble and insoluble fibers like beans and peas, all fruits and vegetables, whole wheat pasta and whole wheat breads. Both soluble and insoluble fiber causes the bowel to traverse the gut more rapidly—33 hours compared to 90 or so hours without it. Soluble fiber therefore, helps prevent as much absorption of fat and cholesterol. Furthermore, magnesium taken with every meal also helps prevent the absorption of cholesterol and fat. You can buy it at the pharmacy but this doesn't mean that you can eat as much fat as you want! **Meat is the number one source of fat in North America. While there's nothing wrong with meat—it's best when you only eat 10% of it for your daily calorie count**—you need to avoid the meat of scavengers like pork at all costs. Too much meat in your diet probably caused your gout in the first place too!

Breast cancer is caused by dietary fat; Dutch women suffer more cases than any in the world due to the fact that they eat lots of fat. Japanese women have the lowest since they eat very little animal fat. Eat more carbohydrates because it burns clean and 20% of its energy is stored as fat. It metabolizes clean and has very few waste products. Choose proper foods and your weight will gradually fall and you'll feel better.

As our body metabolizes fat, one of the waste products produced is estrace. It is a cancer causing estrogenic hormone that is manufactured and reabsorbed to the body and targets sex organs like the breast, the uterus, the ovaries and the prostate. All these different types of cancers of the breast, uterus, ovaries and prostate are all caused by dietary fat. In addition, cancer of the pancreas and several others that we don't have scientific proof as of yet, are also caused by dietary fat and with time science will prove that dietary fat is the villain.

Smoking causes cancer of the lungs. It's a very bad cancer, 10% of the people who get this disease survive this cancer over 5 years and it's completely preventable. If you smoke a pack a day, your risk of lung cancer is 20 times that of a non-smoker. If you smoke 2 packs, your risk is 40 times that of a non-smoker, 3 packs 60 times and 4 packs 80 times! Now put that in your pipe and smoke it! Smoking weakens the immune system by depressing antibodies and cells that protect against foreign invaders. There is an association between smoking and the increased incidence of certain malignant diseases and respiratory infections, according to the National Center for Biotechnology Information (NCBI). There is also a significant decrease in immune cells that normally help the body but this process can be reversed if a smoker gives up the bad habit. Many cancer-causing chemicals from cigarette smoke like carbon monoxide travel throughout the bloodstream and reach the organs of the body, interfere with oxygen levels and damage the immune response. Less oxygen reaches the brain, heart, muscles and other organs and lung functions are reduced because of the narrowing of the airways and presence of excess mucus. Lung irritation and damage result from invading substances leading to infection. Blood pressure and heart rate are affected negatively by smoking chemicals carried through the blood. The immune system does not work as well and smokers become more prone to infections, such as pneumonia and influenza. It takes smokers longer than nonsmokers to get over illnesses. So butt that cigarette out! According to the National Fire Protection Association there are about 140,000 smoking-related fires in the US each year. These fires kill about 900 people and injured more than

2,000 others. This is all preventable by you, go on the nicotine patch, and ask your doctor what other options are available to you to help you quit this habit. In relation to gout, read my post on <u>Gout and Smoking</u>.

So let's do a good recap of what we've learned so far and touch on some other points to get this good information imprinted in our brain. We must eat a very high carbohydrate diet and should consist of 80% of our daily calories. Eat plenty of fruits if you are not diabetic but if you are; limit your daily portion to no more than 3 a day. Another food that causes much confusion from doctors and dieticians is bread, that I want to touch upon. **Fifty percent of your daily calories can come from eating bread.** Bread is called "the staff of life" because it is a very basic food that supports life. The world of bread is vast and varied; some form of bread is found in virtually in every society. Our forefathers lived on it but the big no-no is that we process it to get white flour; <u>we feed the bran of the wheat (the best and healthiest part of the grain) to the hogs</u>. Isn't that stupid?

Eat whole grain pastas, rice, oatmeal barley, corn, beans and peas which are soluble fibers and all legumes and avoid too much absorption of cholesterol and fat. Stay on low protein diet because our need of it is vastly exaggerated and 4 ounces of meat in one day is plenty. Limit your intake of red meat, fish is your best source of protein, it's low on fat and it has plenty of Omega 3 oils which helps drive up our HDL (good cholesterol) and drives down LDL (bad cholesterol). Eating fish 2-3 times a week will decrease our risk of heart disease and risk of heart attack by 50%! Limit your animal fat to avoid coronary heart disease, cancer as well as gout. They say that the main problem of children in Third World countries is protein depletion. But the truth is, their major problem is that they don't get enough calories, so that they burn up their own muscle for energy which is inefficient. If we give them large quantities of grains, vegetables and fruits, they would burn less muscle and require less protein intake.

You can eat as much as you want of anything that has less than 15% of its' calories as fat. For example, corn has as much as 10% of its calories as fat while lettuce stands at 11%, but it doesn't mean that you can go home and eat all of the chicken breast that you want since it has 15% of its calories as fat—don't be a glutton but eat modestly.

There was a study done years ago about the Tarahumara Indians of Mexico who for 2000 years had the same meatless diet, eating primarily sweet potatoes and the vines. A whopping 94% of their calories were carbohydrates and there was never a case of gout, coronary heart disease, colon cancer, breast cancer, ovarian cancer, cancer of the uterus, prostate cancer nor pancreatic cancer—just by that simple diet alone. I'm not suggesting that you go on a sweet potatoes diet but we have known for the past 70 years that the more meat we eat, the lesser our life span will be. Another study done in Papua New Guinea found that the natives ate only carbs with no meat and they also end up with no trace of gout, cancer, heart disease, breast cancer, prostate cancer and so on. Take out your butcher's knife and trim the fat in your meat and barbeque it over fire, to burn away the cholesterol and fat. We live longer if we eat things moderately, but unfortunately we overindulge and then we get into trouble or have a flare-up. Another important lesson is that although drugs may reduce cholesterol by 5-10%, allopurinol may lower uric acid levels, or any other gout drug your doctor has prescribed to you, but the same drugs increase the death rate from other diseases like pancreatitis and gallbladder disease by 36% so be careful of drugs, they do cause damage.

Some stats to share with you here, in men, lung cancer is the number one killer, number two is colon cancer, number three prostate cancer and number four the urinary tract. In women, breast cancer is the number one killer, number two lung cancer, number three colon cancer and number four cancer of the uterus.

Chapter 4:

Preventing High Blood Pressure & Diabetes While Suffering From Gout

Let's now talk about High Blood Pressure which is also a preventable disease. One out three or 77 million adults in the US, about half of them have high blood pressure and it's pretty prevalent. The medical community will tell you that salt is a no-no but it is of no influence in 85% of the people, it only affects people with high blood pressure which consists of only 15%. Am I saying to use all the salt that you want? Of course not, but most people eat too much salt in their diet even though we have no need for it except for the sodium that it contains. What we need, is the sodium that occurs naturally in the food that nature created for us like the fruits, vegetables and grains. They contain all the sodium we really need and we absorb it rapidly. Sodium is a part of everyone's diet, but how much is too much? Under ideal conditions, the minimum sodium requirement is about 1,500 milligrams (mg) per day. This is less than 1 teaspoon of table salt. The maximum recommended level of sodium intake is 2,300 mg per day. On average, American men consume between 3,100 and 4,700 mg of sodium per day, while women consume between 2,300 and 3,100 mg due to their lower caloric intake but not because of sodium restriction.

The standard North American diet is sad; it consists of 40–50% of the calories as fat which should be no more than 10%. If you have a disease like cancer, you must drop all of the fat and be on a 100% strict carbohydrates diet; if you want a chance at reversing your disease. Research has proven that cancer is reversible at certain stages. Studies of breast cancer by the Women's Intervention Nutrition Study (WINS) in 2006 has shown that once patients reduced their fat intake, their cancer decreased in size and responded better to treatment, therefore, the high carb diet works even if you have cancer.

We must understand how cancer comes about. The macrophages, those large white cells which whose job is to digest debris and bacteria, one of the body's main lines of defence, won't work for you if they are filled with fat. We eat a big fatty meal, the fat gets into our bloodstream, the macrophages try to devour it and destroy it because it knows they are not good for your health. The body is trying to save you from the problems you are creating. If you are not eating fat, those same macrophages become active and can devour bacteria and cancer cells as they float throughout the body. People who eat a low fat diet generally live longer even if they have cancer! They are more comfortable, particularly if it involves the vital organs like liver cancer.

The medical profession's answer to high blood pressure is to put you on medicine or prescribed drugs if you prefer, for the rest of your life! They prescribe what they call step-up therapy and they start you on diuretics commonly known as "water pills" to help your body get rid of unneeded water and salt through the urine. If that works, then that's all you have to take but if it doesn't, then they keep the "water pill" going and add two to seven more drugs, just to control your blood pressure! Firstly, the diuretics dehydrate you because they cause you to pass a lot of water, so you must drink a lot of water. In turn this will increase your risk of death from other causes. Remember that pills do not cure high blood pressure, they just treat the symptoms. None of the high blood pressure medicines cure you! Zero!

In my post about diuretics you can read about how patients with high blood pressure increase their chances of developing gout while taking "water pills".

So what happens when you get high blood pressure and it becomes atherosclerosis, that hardening of the blood vessels and the arteries narrowing that supply the kidneys. We can only reverse that and we can, it has been proven on many occasions by altering our lifestyle to eating the proper foods that contain no fat, high carbohydrates, exercise and no smoking. If we take the prescribed drugs we notice many complications; they relieve the symptoms but they decrease the blood flow and they dilate the blood vessels that cause many side effects, most notably death! Kidney function decreases due to the fact that prescribed drugs (diuretics, allopurinol, colchicine etc...) cause 20% of the kidney failures. Remember the point I made earlier that health doesn't come in capsules folks. You can't simply poison yourself into health with drugs called medicine. If you want to cure your high blood pressure, then go on a no fat diet that is high in carbs. It is ok to use a little salt, but most foods have it naturally and they do taste fine without it. But then again, there is nothing wrong with adding a bit of salt for most people. With this decreased blood flow caused by high blood pressure, the kidneys and other vital organs can't get enough nutrients and oxygen. The prescribed drugs for high blood pressure cause 50% of men to become impotent within 2 years. Usually men develop high blood pressure when obese for about 8 years and women after 14 years. Women have a built-in factor that protects them in their hormonal level that we don't understand completely yet but it does occur. So obesity plays a role beloved, it's time to start taking action and change your lifestyle forever.

What results can you get without taking the prescribed drugs from your doctor? What I recommend, and please don't do this on your own, please have your doctor monitor it for 4 to 8 weeks or until you get results! Eighty five percent of you will get results within that 8- week period and during that period please, pretty please don't eat any meat, eggs, cheese, butter and milk. You are not going to be on this diet permanently, just for a short period of time. You will eat only fruits, vegetables, grains, whole grain breads and use olive oil in your baking, all of it that you want. That is if you do bake, if not, make sure to read the ingredients or ask your baker if they used olive oil in their baked goods. In a study in a large number of adults, all they did was decrease the fat only to 10% of calories, so there was no visible fat, all the fat was trimmed and no disease was developed. I am not saying that fat is entirely bad, it insulates the body and cushions the vital organs and we have some 40 billion fat cells in our body. But the fats we ingest is the cause of all these troubles. After 8 weeks, you will be off the medicine and during this period, make sure to check your blood pressure twice a day. Decrease the medicine very slowly with medical advice, have your doctor monitor you, he's going to be surprised at the results you get. Remember, if you reduce your fat intake to 10% of your daily calories, your blood pressure will drop by 10% in 10 days. What about 30% of your daily calories as fat? Then forget it, it won't work. The best treatment is nutrition and having your doctor as your monitor. As for any side effect, they will gradually go down as your medicine is discontinued.

Over 4 ½ million people are rushed to the emergency room every year from prescribed drug problems through drug interactions and bad reactions particularly the combination of drugs and many people are allergic to them. Twenty percent of kidney failures are caused by prescribed drugs that we take and hospital staffs make mistakes every single day providing patients with the wrong medicine.

Let's not make the cure worse than the disease itself! With high blood pressure we have a higher chance of getting a stroke; cerebral paralysis which consists of the chain of nerve cells that runs from the brain, through the spinal cord, out to the muscle called the motor pathway. Normal muscle function requires intact connections all along this motor pathway. Damage at any point reduces the brain's ability to control the muscle's movements. This reduced efficiency causes weakness, also called paresis. Complete loss of communication prevents any willed movement at all. This lack of control is called paralysis. Finally, high blood pressure can result in blood clots, trapped blood can form clots that can narrow (and sometimes block) the arteries. These clots sometimes break off and block vessels and the blood supply to different parts of the body. When this happens, heart attacks or strokes are often the result.

So what can we do about it? A high fiber diet helps remove toxins from the body to avoid high blood pressure and cancer. Don't follow diet programs like the Atkins diet, the Jenny Craig diet, protein diet and so on. The diet industry is polarised around simple debates such as fat vs sugar vs protein because there are huge amounts of money at stake. Farmers, food manufacturers, lobbyists, scientists and authors of diet books need to defend one or other side. Fortunately, you don't need to worry about any of that here, cause I'm providing you with proof, by taking my 60 day blood test challenge so you can see for yourself and putting my money where my mouth is!

Don't force yourself off certain foods rather, eat modestly and you can keep eating a little of everything. Rather than make massive lifestyle changes, why not eat properly for the rest of your life without depriving yourself any of your favourite foods? Eat modest quantities, don't be a glutton and eliminate the fat permanently and you will be healthy permanently and hopefully die of old age.

Diabetes is a disease that is 80% preventable with a proper diet and exercise. Just like gout, it is an old disease that manifested itself since Egyptian times. It is often said that only royalty can afford the "rich" foods like meat, sugar and wine. Gout which is closely related to diabetes is often referred to as "the rich man's disease" or "the disease of kings". You see the peasants ate only fruits, vegetables and grains and the healthy carbohydrates grown from their farms and the peasants were healthier than the nobility. So I hope you have taken notes or printed this e-book and highlighted the key points.

Over 300 years ago, an Englishman discovered sugar in the urine of diabetics and concluded that sugar causes diabetes. It's far from the real truth. It is true that glucose tolerance is important to understanding the disease which is the ability to digest sugars or glucose. However, if we cut out the fat of the diabetic, he quickly regains the ability for the insulin to work. Over 90% of the diabetics have 3 or 4 times as much insulin as they require. It has been rendered inactive, unable to function due to the fat that is absorbed and caused those cells not to function (insulin). If we want glucose tolerance to increase, we must exercise on a daily basis and after 3 or 4 days, its' good effect will already begin to kick in. What are we saying then? The University of Kentucky has proven in a study that if you cut the fat intake to no more than 10% of your daily calories, your diabetes simply goes away! Diabetes is not too hard to cure; you can be cured, even if you have to take insulin within 3 to 5 weeks by removing the fat from your diet. There are over 10 million diabetics in the US and over half of them are not diagnosed. According to the International Diabetes Federation there are 371 million people that have diabetes globally and about half are undiagnosed. Already, $471 billion was spent treating the disease in 2012, up $6 billion from last year. In the U.S. alone, $174 billion was spent in 2007 to combat diabetes, according to the American Diabetes Association. I know many different more productive ways to spend $471 billion dollars than helping to find a cure for diabetes. The cure is so simple, that a child can understand!

Seventy percent of these people are obese and heart disease occurs 3 times as often in diabetics! Do you want me to scare you some more? Eighty percent of the amputations due to gangrene are directly linked to diabetes. Gangrene is the result of severely impaired blood flow to parts of the body. In some cases, the affected part of the body must be surgically removed to prevent further medical problems. Amputation is a last-resort treatment for gangrene, but it can be life-saving. Most amputations are performed on the toe, foot, arm or leg. Seventy percent of new blindness cases come from diabetics. Over ninety percent of diabetics have 3 or 4 times the amount of insulin that they need. As fat enters the bloodstream, the platelets become sensitive and insensitive and they can't burn simple sugars. Does that mean we have to remove carbohydrates? No, but conventional wisdom says yes. If you exercise and continue to eat complex carbohydrates by avoiding simple sugars completely, you will do well; you can't eat all the fruit you want because the fruit is actually a complex carbohydrate that has a lot of sugar in it. Diabetics can't metabolize large quantities of them, eat a limit of 3 portions a day if you are diabetic and that doesn't mean you can eat peaches in syrup! Use common sense, eat only fresh fruits! <u>This is not a hereditary disease but in medical schools it is taught that it is</u>. An English professor studied 300 sets of twins and some of them had diabetes and the other one has gone on for more than 30 years and still doesn't have it! So it is not hereditary, we are talking about identical twins here! Avoid the confusion from the media and other so called "health experts". **Walk 3 miles a day and eat the proper foods outlined to you from this e-book and you will see results.**

Cromolyn is very good, its role is to maintain glucose tolerance and provide that ability for the body to digest these complex carbohydrates and simple sugars. It also brings down cholesterol a little bit. Certainly, go on brewer's yeast which has plenty of cromolyn in it, it won't cure you but then again do drugs cure you? No they don't, they just relieve the symptoms and you can become diabetic very quickly if you eat the wrong things. There are 250% more deaths among diabetics who are treated for their diabetes with drugs instead of nutrition. Imagine that! Yet 85% of cardiologists continue to treat diabetes with drugs! Focus on quality foods instead, regardless of what the American Heart Association and American Diabetes Association have to say on the matter. They simply have not taken enough fat out of the diet to do us any good. You will need to be treated with drugs for the rest of your life! A good experiment to do is to lay a paper towel down and put a piece of cheese on it, then set it out in the hot sun around noontime on a summer day for a couple of hours. Then bring it in to see how much fat has been bled out of it. **So the question remains, are we victims of all these diseases or do we bring it on ourselves? The answer is simple; we bring it on ourselves from what we eat.** "Well I thought my uncle John had it and that I will develop it too!" you might say. Your uncle John had the same bad habits that you also developed, probably by watching him and allowed it to happen to you! Discipline yourself! Avoid the fat! And exercise!

Gout sufferers also have an increased risk of developing diabetes since both diseases are linked, you can read more about it on my post titled Gout and Diabetes.

Many of us now have jobs that don't require a lot of physical exertion and as a result we don't get the exercise we need. If you go back just over a century ago, most of us were living in rural areas, working laboriously on farms. Obesity wasn't an issue, our bodies are meant to move, walk, lift and not sit in one position for 8 hours in a day. Then go home to sit or lie down on the couch for another couple of hours. Let's conclude that diabetes is curable, preventable and we know the cause, so let's do something about it. If you suffer from diabetes, don't forget to have your doctor monitor you should you wish to go off the drugs as I have repeated many times before.

Chapter 5:

What Foods Can We Eat In A Gout Diet Plan & To Prevent Other Diseases?

We hear in the news all the time about health care and Obamacare but have we stopped to ask if we need more health care? The answer is we do not need more health care; we just need more health advice.

Remember that cooks are the guardians of your health. They are the ones that stand between you eating and them preparing and cooking the food. This is a big responsibility, so watch out who cooks and prepares your meals at home or at any restaurant you eat at. What I want you to do is to develop your own recipes and start taking the fat out of your diet. Start by removing 50% of the fat then gradually reduce it to 75% until you can manage eating with only 10% of your daily calories as fat. Make it a family thing whereby each member contributes to the meals either by helping the preparation and cooking or researching and suggesting a new recipe. This e-book has over 100 recipes to get you started and all the meals are delicious. Now let's look closely at a study done by Jim Anderson from the University of Kentucky. What he did was take 20 people under hospital condition and he fed them oatmeal, some everyday for a period of 3 weeks. He began with people who had blood cholesterol of 280, a very high blood cholesterol level since the average blood cholesterol level when you have a heart attack is about 140! He found that the blood cholesterol went down by 13% and if we equate this with the risk of coronary heart disease, the risk goes down twice as much or 26% in 3 weeks. Then came along another study from Harvard University wiz's, a supposed "good" university and basically this research was primarily done to confuse you or muddy the water. The researcher started with people who had blood cholesterol of 186 and he fed them oatmeal also and it did nothing for them. This is plain stupid because their blood cholesterol level was already normal before he started, so there was no absolute need to have it reduced and obviously it reduced very little! The other study started with people who had blood cholesterol level of 200 and again it didn't need dropping either, so obviously it didn't drop very much. As a result of these studies, they have caused confusion everywhere and your health depends on it.

Jim Anderson is one of the few researchers that understands that if you drop fat to 10% of your caloric intake, that your diabetes will simply go away. Feed yourself a carbohydrate diet and exercise; and diabetes will go away! The key then is to eat no fat with cholesterol in it and your cholesterol will drop at least by 25% in 3 to 4 weeks. By doing this, you also reduce the risk of heart attack by 50% in a very short period of time and this is without taking any medicine. For gout sufferers you will see a notable decrease in your uric acid levels and no gout attacks! Fat is the villain, the bad guy, the evil empire looking to invade and destroy your entire body!

Beans have more protein than any other food including meat! Isn't that interesting? Whole grain breads have more protein per calorie than meat does, so naturally bread is a good source or protein that gives you that "full feeling". Remember, that we can eat 50% of our daily calories as bread. **Range beef** has 9% of its calories as fat since it has less marbling; it is tougher but a better source of meat than other beefs. If the meat is very lean, it can have one third as much fat as a similar cut from a grain-fed animal. But a diet high in protein can potentially kill you! Meat-eating societies have a much shorter life span. A good example of this is the Eskimos, where their average life span is approximately 50 years or so.

Today's animal meat is full of growth hormones, antibiotics, pesticides, herbicides, nuclear wastes, high levels of adrenaline, and other toxic chemicals from air and ground pollution. All of these compounds are considered carcinogenic or cancer-causing. We find more cancer in the cows, pigs and chickens today, than ever before. And man eats this! We have also lost our integrity and sense of decency. Many farmers are now grinding up their sick and dying cows, pigs and chickens and mixing this "dead" often "diseased" meat into their regular animal feeds. This leads to "mad cow" and "hoof and mouth" disease. We see this now, especially in Europe where they have been feeding dead sheep meat to living cows. Cows are vegetarians; and hogs are not true meat eaters, either. This eventually leads to acidosis and disease within these animals, just as it does within us. Meat eating is known to be one of the chief and most direct causes of tooth decay. Let's look at a study quoted in the NY Times on March 12, 2012:

"Eating red meat is associated with a sharply increased risk of death from cancer and heart disease, according to a new study, and the more of it you eat, the greater the risk. The analysis, published online Monday in Archives of Internal Medicine, used data from two studies that involved 121,342 men and women who filled out questionnaires about health and diet from 1980 through 2006. There were 23,926 deaths in the group, including 5,910 from cardiovascular disease and 9,464 from cancer.

People who ate more red meat were less physically active and more likely to smoke and had a higher body mass index, researchers found. Still, after controlling for those and other variables, they found that each daily increase of three ounces of red meat was associated with a 12 percent greater risk of dying over all, including a 16 percent greater risk of cardiovascular death and a 10 percent greater risk of cancer death.

The increased risks linked to processed meat, like bacon, were even greater: 20 percent overall, 21 percent for cardiovascular disease and 16 percent for cancer. If people in the study had eaten half as much meat, the researchers estimated, deaths in the group would have declined 9.3 percent in men and 7.6 percent in women. Previous studies have linked red meat consumption and mortality, but the new results suggest a surprisingly strong link.

"When you have these numbers in front of you, it's pretty staggering," said the study's lead author, Dr. Frank B. Hu, a professor of medicine at Harvard."

You want more proof, here you go: A 2007 study of more than 35,000 women published in the British Journal of Cancer found that women who ate the most meat had the highest risk of breast cancer. One study compared cancer rates of vegetarians and meat-eaters in 34,000 Americans. The results showed that those who avoided meat, fish, and poultry had dramatically lower rates of prostate, ovarian, and colon cancer compared to meat-eaters. A study comparing the dietary habits of men in 32 countries found that the highest risk factors for prostate cancer mortality were meat and dairy products. By contrast, another study of men diagnosed with prostate cancer showed that a diet rich in fruits, vegetables, and grains can slow or even halt the progression of the disease. Scientists from the Bremen Institute for Prevention, Research, and Social Medicine and the German Cancer Research Center observed in the American Journal of Clinical Nutrition that "the relationship between a vegetarian and fiber-rich diet and a decreased risk for colon cancer has been reported in many studies." What is the lesson we all learned? A high protein diet can kill you; don't fall for that idiotic Atkins diet or other stupid fads, be smarter, educate yourself and pat yourself on the back on a job well-done by purchasing this e-book! I hope this e-book helped you dig in your brain and take out all the junk information, knowledge and deceptions you have acquired over the years and filled it up with some good old fashioned common sense.

Carbohydrates have 4 calories per gram and remember to eat 80% of your calories as carbs and you can do fine with even more because it is pure energy. We have learned from athletes that we increase our endurance by 3 times just by adding a carbohydrate diet through our exercise regime. The liver and muscles, as we begin to exercise, begin to store carbs in the form of glycogen (glucose). For immediate energy, as we store this carb, it then gives you energy and you feel good.

For children less than 2 years of age, do not place fat restrictions on them because fat provides them with the building blocks for the body particularly that cholesterol from milk. Do not worry about the fat they eat, after the age of 2, you can start placing restrictions. Seventy five percent of American children are too fat because they eat too much junk food. Use common sense and cut back reasonably. Be a good example on the kitchen table so they can see what you eat and they can do likewise. Sixty eight percent of children eat too much salt and we don't need any salt, we need sodium from the fruits, vegetables and grains that we eat. Many of our children have high blood cholesterol; about 46% of them have high blood pressure although they are below 15 years age. Health is the greatest wealth, don't eat yourself to death but eat for a healthier you!

Disease is a major factor in the world today. The number one factor is chronic poisoning from eating too much fat and protein and we are poisoning ourselves. Number two is malnutrition; eating too much fat and sugar, neither of which has any nutrients in them, however, they do have many empty calories and they don't help your immune system by preventing diseases. Hippocrates, the father of medicine said: **"Let your food be thy medicine and let your medicine be your food."** We haven't really progressed as much as we think we have, in spite of our knowledge, we have failed completely in the prevention of disease! We have learned and pored many dollars on research on how to handle the problem once it occurs instead of prevention which is the key. Universities and medical schools spend little time teaching doctors how to prevent diseases; you must take responsibility for yourself. People need health advice and not more health care.

What are some of the worst foods to eat? Soda pop is up there with 10 teaspoons of sugar in every can, you can see why! For gout sufferers read my post on sugar and high fructose corn syrup. Fruit juice is better but be careful, don't overdo it! French fries is a travesty on the name of "potato", as we fry them, they soak up 200 calories of nothing but fat! A potato is good for you but not if you fry it! Chips are virtually all fat and worse than fries! Bacon, 95% of its calories are fat! Fettuccine Alfredo and other pasta sauces are swimming in a pool of grease and destroy the value that you would get from pasta, the only part that is good! Use a no-oil Italian dressing or olive oil instead and you won't have any trouble. Fast food burgers are bad news since half of the calories are fat anyway. I'm not telling you not to eat beef, but in moderation please and don't dress it up with fat, like cheese and sauces. How about granola bars? They are horrible and are promoted as a health food but they're half fat and the other half all sugar, no worse than a candy bar! Donuts are very bad for you, cheese is ok to eat, eat it with meat or replace meat with it instead but don't think cheese is a wonder food, be moderate. Hot dogs are definitely not good for you since 85% of the calories are fat. Candy bars are 50–50 fat and sugar, please eat it only once in a while even for your children. It also keeps your bank savings higher by not dishing out big bucks in getting their teeth fixed by the dentist.

Some of the best foods are broccoli and carrots loaded with vitamin A; a precursor of beta-carotene that helps prevent cancer. All fruits and vegetables have something to prevent cancer, so eat plenty of it! Oats are great, baked potatoes are fantastic, yogurt and skim milk are good, fish which has very little fat and helps prevent blood clots, whole grain breads are outstanding, lentils and other dried beans are extraordinary, popcorn and bananas with their high energy! In conclusion, there is no miracle food out there, just eat a variety of the good foods and you will live very well!

In your gout diet plan make sure to eat cherries which lowers uric acid levels, fruits and vegetables that are high in Vitamin C like oranges, kiwis, peppers, kale, broccoli, berries and tomatoes. Pineapple is a gout favorite, studies have found that bromelain is useful in relieving strain-induced gout, when uric acid crystals accumulate in a joint that becomes inflamed by a strain or even normal use. Bromelain causes the uric acid crystals to decompose thus relieving you from the pain associated with gout. Unlike pineapple stems, pineapple fruit does not contain enough bromelain enzyme to provide any provable medicinal effects. If taken regularly, bromelain may also prevent repeated gout attacks. Foods high in potassium like bananas are also key in order to reduce uric acid levels. Make sure to favor these certain foods over others since they are more beneficial for your uric acid levels in avoiding gout attacks in the future. Yes I also use apple cider vinegar in my salads, occasionally cook with turmeric, have some celery seeds, flax seeds and sprinkle some cinnamon in my oatmeal but there is no one single remedy in beating gout, you have to follow a healthy gout diet plan where your diet consists of 80% carbohydrates, 10% fat, 10% protein and some exercise. There is no magic potion in a bottle either! All those snake oil salesmen on the web who try to sell you their brand of a gout cure are simply robbing you blind. Ya, you could probably take some baking soda relieve yourself of a gout attack once or twice but it won't cure you...You can't take a home remedy and say to yourself, that you can eat all the junk that you want. Good gout health can only come from the diet I just described to you in this e-book...Nothing else! This is also true for all diseases not just gout, as you have read in this e-book from the other diseases I've touched upon. All these diseases are caused due to our bad eating habits and lack of exercise. It's that simple. By following this diet, your body will also adjust and become more alkaline. Many web sites with information about the alkaline diet also sell courses, books, supplements, and alkaline-infused water, food, and drinks. You do not need to buy these things to follow the alkaline diet. The Gout Diet Plan in this e-book is alkaline, so I saved you hundreds if not thousands of dollars in the process.

What if you are obese and have gout? The next paragraph is verbatim from my post on weight loss:

It's not a big revelation that being obese or being above your ideal weight can cause you a lot of health problems and one of them of course is gout. When I got my first gout attack I weighed 240 pounds, about 45 pounds overweight from my ideal weight as per my doctor.

I had what is called central obesity, basically carrying weight around my middle, having a pot belly if you prefer.

Losing weight alone can decrease uric acid levels in the blood, as well as the number of gout attacks, staving off hyperuricemia, so it's a no brainer that if you are overweight and have gout that you immediately consider losing weight with whatever method you like. In addition, weight loss will also help relieve your joints (knees, feet, hips, ankles etc...) by reducing the stress from the excessive weight, avoiding pain in those joints.

If you are determined to lose weight, it is important that you avoid crash dieting at all costs since rapid weight loss as well as going hungry for long periods of time will increase uric acid levels in your body and cause you a gout attack. A balanced diet rich in fruits and vegetables, with low meat intake, plenty of whole wheat bread, whole wheat cereals, moderate amounts of dairy products, plenty of water, little alcohol if any at all, the complete elimination of highly processed foods and drinks is the key to a successful gout diet. This will help you control your weight and provide you with all the necessary nutrients required for you to fight this disease.

The famous gout researcher Hyon K. Choi from Massachusetts General Hospital while studying 47 150 middle aged men for a period of 12 years did conclude that the more weight men gained the more susceptible they were in getting a gout attack or developing the disease. Those who did lose weight though decreased their gout risk especially weight loss of more than 10 pounds, dropping their risk by 40%. Choi also concluded that regardless of their diet, men who gained weight would get gout more often. Overweight men with a BMI (Body Mass Index) of at least 25 are more than twice as likely to develop gout and obese men have triple the risk in developing it!

Another small pilot study on gout and weight loss was done with 13 gout patients, while all 13 were gout patients who would get an attack every month and after losing weight through their diet after a few months only but one patient would have less than one gout attack per month. Yet another study conducted at the University of Auckland in New Zealand also suggests that gout patients who are obese may benefit from bariatric surgery which will result in lowering uric acid crystallization in the joints further preventing gout attacks and reduced inflammation from the weight loss.

Weight loss allows the uric acid in the fatty deposits inside the body to leave or excrete in a consistent manner. If you have a gout attack or swelling in any of your joints, it will help diminish those effects due to the fact there will be less fatty deposits in your joints knees, toes, feet etc... If you plan on losing weight, make sure you are losing 1-2 pounds a week and not more avoiding increasing your uric acid levels abruptly causing a painful gout attack. So tread carefully and do it right!

If you don't have gout make sure to maintain a healthy weight in order to avoid getting it. Weight loss is not the only answer when it comes to curing your gout but it is a big piece in the overall pie, that's for sure. Remember to begin with small changes in the beginning making sure you are losing only 1-2 pounds a week in order to avoid a gout attack, then keep progressing in eliminating whatever foods that are bad for you for healthier choices eventually moving towards your ideal weight. Don't forget to include your doctor's advice when planning your diet, even consulting with a dietitian can do wonders.

By following the Gout Diet Plan from this e-book as well as my recommendation to exercise, you will drop the pounds in a natural and healthy way avoiding a painful gout attack. Weight loss cannot be done quickly or extremely when you have gout cause you will pay the price by suffering an attack, so eat right as outlined in my e-book and you'll drop the weight in no time. Remember for exercise, if you don't want to do anything more strenuous you can simply walk 3 miles a day and it'll do the trick.

Now let's talk a little about alcohol. When it comes to gout, you need to totally avoid it if I were you, or limit it to an ounce or 2 of hard liquor once in a while, 1-2 beers max or 1-2 glasses of wine on occasions like a wedding, party, BBQ and so on. If you do drink make sure to drink lots and I mean lots of water that day. For more information on <u>Gout and Alcohol</u>, please read my post.

Yes, studies have proven that a very moderate intake of alcohol mostly red wine can cut your risk of heart disease but they kill another way. Fifty percent of fatal car accidents are caused by alcohol. A couple drinks of 2 ounces of whisky a day decrease the heart's workload capacity by 20%. It's no secret that alcohol consumption can cause major health problems, including cirrhosis of the liver and injuries sustained in automobile accidents. But if you think liver disease and car crashes are the only health risks posed by drinking, think again: researchers have linked alcohol consumption to more than 60 diseases.

"Alcohol does all kinds of things in the body, and we're not fully aware of all its effects," says James C. Garbutt, MD, professor of psychiatry at the University of North Carolina at Chapel Hill School of Medicine and a researcher at the university's Bowles Center for Alcohol Studies. "It's a pretty complicated little molecule."

Here are 12 conditions linked to chronic heavy drinking: anemia, cancer, cardiovascular disease, cirrhosis of the liver, dementia, depression, seizures, gout, high blood pressure, infectious diseases, nerve damage and pancreatitis. (Source www.webmd.com) So again beloved, please drink moderately, do not get drunk and more importantly do not drink and drive.

Take care of that temple, your flesh body in health. There are approximately 13 million alcoholics in this country and concerning women who are pregnant and drink an alcoholic beverage, the fetus will have the same blood alcohol level as with the pregnant woman within 15 minutes! If you drink excessively or even moderately, it can potentially create big problems for the child like having a lesser birth weight and you more apt to miscarry. So try and avoid alcohol if you can.

Chapter 6:

A word about Tophi

Tophus or Tophi in plural is the same thing but what exactly is it? In Latin it is defined as a stone. Ouch! You know this post won't be pretty! Very simply, it is a deposit in the elbow, toe, ankle, knee, ear, fingers or other joint in the body of monosodium urate crystals in people who've had high uric acid levels of over 6-7mg/dl for a prolonged period of time, a stage of gout's development called chronic tophaceous gout. With time a tophus will grow and go unnoticed but then it will grow and bunch up together into bigger lumps of many tophi. Overall, 25% of gout suffers actually have tophi to some extent. Hard to believe that there wasn't an actual treatment for it until 1951 when the drug *phobenecid* was first introduced. What did gout sufferers do before that?

Tophi should not be ignored when it first appears, although painless at the beginning, if left untreated the condition will worsen as they cluster together and more uric acid crystals form around the lump. What happens is our white blood cells attack the invading uric acid crystals so what tophi really is then is a collection of crystals and dead cells. This is not usually painful until they break out from the skin and appear as white or yellowish chalky lumps. It can cause havoc to one's health by destroying the joints, cartilage and harming the organs (complications such as kidney stones) leading to noticeable disabilities.

Without any treatment, tophi can appear on average at about 10 years after being first diagnosed with gout but can develop earlier in older people although they can first appear anywhere between 3 and 42 years! In addition, tophi can appear or pop up suddenly overnight and sometimes the lump may actually grow so big that it must be amputated in order for the joint to be free to move again. This can also cause the tophi sufferer to end up getting an artificial joint. Furthermore, tophi usually appears in the coldest parts of the body in areas furthest from the heart and where obviously blood circulation is the poorest hence the appearance in the toes, ears, fingers and ankles.

The symptoms of tophi include chronic joint pain and the visible lump in the joint, while the pain may be mild and include some inflammation but in many cases, tophi is usually painless and may cause only stiffness of the joints. On a sidenote, tophi can grow into the bones as well on top of them!

One thing is for sure, it is very difficult to treat tophi with a simple change in diet but you can definitely lower your risk of developing tophi by following a low purine diet avoiding too much meat, seafood, alcohol, sugars and drinking a lot of water, keeping those uric acid levels on the low end of the spectrum. Tophi's growth can be stopped and beginning to dissolve when the uric acid blood levels begin reaching 6mg/dl and below but the majority of the time when tophi has formed, medical intervention is required, usually they are surgically removed. There is also the drug Krystexxa which can shrink the tophi quickly which is a modern uricase treatment, as well as febuxostat (EU brand name Adenuric, US brand name Uloric).

Prevention is the key to avoiding tophi in your lifetime while suffering from gout. Make sure to live a healthy lifestyle of a good gout diet, exercise, no smoking and following your doctor's recommendations and you will be fine. Tophi is definitely not something you want to develop later on. Please follow my Gout Diet Plan and stick to it, do not deviate from the plan!

Chapter 7:

Big Pharma and the

Greedy Food Companies

I added this chapter so you the reader can clearly understand why there is so much confusion in regards what to and what not to eat, why there is so much contradictory information about fat, protein, sugar and carbohydrates and how big Pharma and the greedy food companies all care about is profit. At the end the confusion helps their bottom line, as long as you don't know the truth and you get sick, there is profit to be made.

We have all heard or read of stories involving drug companies and some of the horrible offences they commit as corporate citizens. On an episode of Dr. Oz aired on May 12, 2011, Dr. Oz interviewed author of "Overdosed America" Dr. John Abramson and author of the book "Drug Truths" Dr. LaMattina exposing drug companies on what they don't want you to know like controlling much of the information your doctor gets about a drug, how you are often prescribed drugs that you simply don't need. I have discussed in this e-book, how drugs target the symptoms and not the actual cause of your health problem. Beloved, it is only common sense that a drug company's real purpose is to sell drugs in order to earn profit for its shareholders, so ethics will take a back seat to greed and corruption and this is human nature. Furthermore, we are a nation obsessed with taking pills. For example, with the weight loss drugs Alli and Xenical, there's an ingredient called "Orlistat" which the FDA is being pressured to take out of the market. Orlistat has been linked to severe liver disease, acute pancreatic damage and kidney stones.

Then you have wilder claims as quoted by Dr. Adriane Fugh-Berman Director of PharmedOut that "pharmaceutical companies actually invented specific diseases or conditions and it's not only diseases that have been invented, but categories have been changed. Anytime a disease category is expanded it increases the number of people who are eligible for drug treatment. Right now much of the prescribing in the United States is not rational, people are being prescribed drugs where the risks outweigh the benefits." You're often prescribed drugs you don't need. Dr. Oz says that drug companies are inventing diseases and it's called disease mongering, hyping up conditions that really aren't diseases. You see these in commercials about overactive bladder, osteopenia, excessive daytime sleepiness etc. They are problems but do they really need drugs in order to be treated? Dr. Abramson said this is a widespread practice in the industry, the drug industry's job is to sell drugs, they get the drugs approved on the market for an indication that is truly helpful and then broaden the marketing so that you get to a much greater population of people who are a candidate for the drug.

When it comes to the side effects, many drugs have life threatening risks associated with them, Dr. Abramson stated: "the drug companies own the data, it's like their playing poker and they can see the cards and they don't have to show it to the doctors, they don't have to show it to the consumers, they often don't even show it to the authors of the articles – evidence in the journals that doctors trust." (Now that is scary!) Dr. Abramson said almost all the information that the doctors have and the consumers have is coming directly or indirectly from the drug companies. About 85% of clinical trials are funded by the drug industry and they own the data like Coca-Cola owns the recipe for Coke. So the doctors don't understand that they're getting a selected and filtered version of what the information is. On the subject of antidepressant medications, Dr. Abramson said evidence has shown these drugs have increased suicidal thinking in kids and young adults. So we're getting no benefit but all risks.

The plain truth is that most prescription drugs are nothing more than a counterfeit of the same thing offered in nature, as evidenced by the testimony of Dr. Edwin Cooper, professor at the University of California. He states that several valuable drugs have been derived from parts of plant and animal sources, including aspirin, anti-cancer agents, anti-psychotics and antibiotics. For gout sufferers, colchicine is derived from the plant called *Colchicum* also known as "autumn crocus" or "meadow saffron". Yet the big drug companies, whose profits are reaching historical levels, don't want you to know this for rather obvious reasons. People taking natural remedies would hit the drug pusher's profits hard, but they brought that mistrust on themselves. Excessive drug cost to consumers is forcing people to look for alternative cures. A case in point; the mysterious bird flu scare that caused such mass hysteria. The people were scared into seeking the preventive measure that would inoculate the dreaded symptoms. Do you think the pharmaceutical company, Roche, made a few bucks on the deal? Tamiflu earned them over $2 billion.

It is in your hands only, to eat right, exercise and not get sick later on. You are responsible! It's not for your doctor and the money-hungry drug companies to make a significant lifestyle change with your diet. It is in the drug companies' best financial interest to just mask and maintain the symptoms so they can continue making money off you unto your last breath! Even congressman Ron Paul from Texas has made the admission to the public on tape that the FDA and Big Pharma are indeed "in bed together" both building up their monopolies and only interested in making more money. Big Pharma loves government medicine because they make more money. He's been quoted as saying: "The insurance companies and the drug companies, whether it's Democrats or Republicans reforming the medical care system, these corporations run the show. You know, they support it, it's because the government doesn't take it over. It's the corporations that end up taking over."

Drug reps often have no medical or science education. Is it safe for physicians to assume that the professionals they meet with to discuss new medications and prescription recommendations for their patients actually have backgrounds in medicine or science? According to ABC News, it's not. A former drug rep for the pharmaceutical company Eli Lily, Shahram Ahari testified before Congress, saying that "pharmaceutical companies hire former cheerleaders and ex-models to wine and dine doctors, exaggerate the drug's benefits and underplay their side-effects." He also explained that he was taught "how to exceed spending limits for important clients...[by] using friendships and personal gifts" and to "exploit sexual tension."

Your healthcare provider may have an ulterior motive behind your prescription. In 2007, the St. Petersburg Times reported that drug reps often give gifts to convince medical professionals to prescribe the medications that they represent. Dr. James P. Orlowski tries to teach his students that interaction with drug reps is not in the best interests of patients. Even though many doctors may believe solicitation from drug reps is unethical or at the very least impractical, gifts like free meals, pens, posters, books, and free samples are offered to physicians in an effort to influence their prescription practices.

Pharmaceutical companies spend more on marketing than research. According to Science Daily, a "new study by two York University researchers estimates the U.S. pharmaceutical industry spends almost twice as much on promotion as it does on research and development." Despite pharmaceutical companies' claims that Americans pay such high prices for prescription medications because they're really paying for research and development costs, the industry spent $33.5 billion on promotion costs in 2004. The study also "supports the position that the U.S. pharmaceutical industry is marketing-driven and challenges the perception of a research-driven, life-saving, pharmaceutical industry" that values the lives of its patients, rather than their spending habits.

What is sad is that Americans pay more for prescription meds than anyone else in the world. The Media Matters website analyzes a *60 Minutes* interview between correspondent Bob Simon and then Surgeon General Richard H. Carmona. During the segment, Carmona maintains that Americans pay more for brand name prescriptions than anyone else in the world because of the hefty price associated with "the research and development of drugs." Americans spent $200 billion on prescription drugs in 2002: Marcia Angell reveals in her book *"The Truth About the Drug Companies"* that Americans spent $200 billion on prescription drugs in 2002. That's the amount medical experts estimated it will cost to rebuild New Orleans after Hurricane Katrina, and the amount China is pouring into an energy renewal program.

Some drug companies are taking advantage of underdeveloped countries to perform clinical trials. Wired.com reports that India is becoming a more attractive place for drug companies to run clinical trials and test out new drugs. The article explains, "more and more drug companies are conducting clinical trials in developing countries where government oversight is more lax and research can be done for a fraction of the cost." Controversy is starting to build over the trend, however, as one expert explains. Sean Philpott, managing editor of The American Journal of Bioethics, reveals to Wired.com that such practices may be unfair, as "individuals who participate in Indian clinical trials usually won't be educated. Offering $100 [as payment for their participation] may be undue enticement; they may not even realize that they are being coerced."

Finally, good PR trumps patient care: When Merck & Co. found out that one of their products, Vioxx, can increase the risk of heart attacks in its patients, it allegedly "played down" the evidence. Cleveland Clinic cardiologist Dr. Eric Topol accused Merck of "scientific misconduct," and two days later, Dr. Topol was kicked off the board of governors at the Cleveland Clinic.

Watch out beloved when a doctor prescribes you a drug. Make sure to do your research on it by checking references online, speaking to others who have taken the drug on online forums and asking another doctor for a second opinion. Remember that your health is at stake and you are responsible for its consequences to your body. Educate yourself beforehand and you won't be sorry!

Who else is making us sick? The food companies of course. We couldn't resist leaving them behind! Check out these sobering stats: In the U.S., four companies pack 83.5% of beef and 66% of pork, and crush 80% of soybeans. Two companies sell 58% of all U.S. seed corn. Corporations produce 98% of poultry in the U.S. In 2006, farms larger than 2,000 acres made up 7% of all farms receiving government aid, but they got 26% of the money. In 1935, the average farm was 135 acres. In 2002, average was 441 acres, median was 2,190. 2% of farms produce 50% of all agricultural products in the country. U.S. farmers use 2 billion kg of pesticides per year. Worldwide use is 10 billion kg. Genetically engineered herbicide resistant crops have led to a 122- million pound increase in pesticide use. In 2000, 25% of corn and 54% of soybeans grown in the U.S. were genetically modified. In 2008, the numbers were 80% and 92%. Iceberg lettuce, frozen and fried potatoes, potato chips, and canned tomatoes make up almost half of U.S. vegetable consumption. In 1967, U.S. per capita consumption of high fructose corn syrup was 0.03 pounds per year. In 2006, it was 58.2. Total consumption of all sweeteners went up 23% in the same period. 75% of the world's food is generated from just 12 varieties of plants and five animal species. In 2007, before the current recession, 36.2 million people in the U.S. lived in food insecure households, including 12.4 million children. Global food prices increased almost 50% in 2008. Americans generate roughly 30 million tons of food waste each year. Sixty six percent of adult Americans are overweight or obese.

A great article posted on www.preventioninstitute.org talks about the facts of junk food marketing and kids:

"The food, beverage, and chain restaurant industries say they're on the side of health, but their actions show otherwise. Experts agree that junk food is a huge contributor to skyrocketing rates of diabetes, high blood pressure, and even strokes. And food and beverage companies spend billions of dollars promoting unhealthy foods virtually everywhere kids go. The Interagency Working Group on Foods Marketed to Children (IWG) has proposed reasonable nutrition guidelines to help provide a model for companies that market to kids. Unfortunately, the food industry and media companies are working to get Congress to stop the IWG from finalizing these sensible recommendations."

Read the facts below and watch "We're Not Buying It," a video that exposes deceptive marketing to children, debunks industry claims, and highlights the latest research. When we put children first, the plan of action is clear: companies should market the foods that keep kids healthy, not sugary cereals and other junk food. The IWG guidelines will help to do just that.

The food, beverage, and chain restaurant industry is targeting our children with intensive junk food marketing:

- The food and beverage industry spends approximately $2 billion per year marketing to children.
- The fast food industry spends more than $5 million every day marketing unhealthy foods to children.
- Kids watch an average of over ten food-related ads every day (nearly 4,000/year).
- Ad spending for interactive video games is projected to reach $1 billion by 2014, with six million 3–11 year olds visiting some form of virtual game online each month.
- Nearly all (98%) of food advertisements viewed by children are for products that are high in fat, sugar or sodium. Most (79%) are low in fiber.

And it's working

- Nearly 40% of children's diets come from added sugars and unhealthy fats.
- Only 21% of youth age 6–19 eat the recommended five or more servings of fruits and vegetables each day.
- A mere 12% of grains consumed by children are whole.

- One study found that when children were exposed to television content with food advertising, they consumed 45% more food than children exposed to content with non-food advertising.

The food and beverage industry may say they're on the side of health, but their actions show otherwise:

- A 2011 review found that "company pledges to reduce food marketing of unhealthy products have failed to protect children <12 years for all types of marketing practices promoting such foods".
- Additionally, in 2010, an independent study documented that only 12 of 3039 children's meal combinations in fast food chain restaurants met established nutrition criteria for preschoolers; only 15 meals met nutrition criteria for older children.
- Each day, African–American children see twice as many calories advertised in fast-food commercials as White children.
- In 2010, the food and beverage industry spent over $40 billion lobbying congress against several regulations including those that would decrease the marketing of unhealthy foods to kids, and potential soda taxes.
- A study conducted by Prevention Institute in 2007, found that over half of the most aggressively marketed children's foods advertising fruit on the packaging actually contain no fruit ingredients whatsoever.
- In 2011, a second study by researchers at Prevention Institute looked at packages with front of package labelling–symbols that identify healthier products–and found that 84% of products studied didn't meet basic nutritional standards.

If we continue on this path, the future health of our children is not so bright:

- Even five years after children have been exposed to promotions of unhealthy foods, researchers found that they purchased fewer fruits, vegetables and whole grains, but increased their consumption of fast foods, fried foods and sugar-sweetened beverages.
- According to the CDC, if current trends continue, 1 of 3 U.S. adults will have diabetes by 2050.
- By 2030, healthcare costs attributable to poor diet and inactivity could range from $860 billion to $956 billion, which would account for 15.8 to 17.6% of total healthcare costs, or one in every six dollars spent on healthcare.

You can see the reason why you probably developed gout in the first place. It all started while you were a toddler, eating the garbage that you and your parents were marketed to. It's all about the money folks! Like pharmaceutical companies, a food company's primary goal is to make as much money and profit as possible. I strongly recommend that you watch the 2008 documentary film directed by Emmy Award winning filmmaker Robert Kenner *Food, Inc*. The film examines corporate farming in the United States, concluding that agribusiness produces food that is unhealthy, in a way that is environmentally harmful and abusive of both animals and employees. It's a real eye opener on the industry as a whole and its profit-driven practices. Just look at all the news stories from the past few years about the tainted meat scandals causing numerous deaths across North America! Need I say more?

Let's face it, government health recommendations and regulations relating to diet and health have failed miserably. Leading a common sense, healthy lifestyle is your best bet to produce a healthy body and mind, and increase your longevity. Unfortunately, the pharmaceutical industry, the food industry, and even government itself sure won't make it easy for you to avoid the garbage that ruins your health. While spending twice as much on healthcare per capita, we're not getting results. I believe we'll keep seeing more of the same until or unless we change our stance on what a healthy diet is, and what constitutes a healthy lifestyle. We need to move away from the idea that being on a dozen medications means you're doing something right for your health—this is not health care. This is disease management, and it comes at a very steep price, namely your longevity.

Until or unless the US government takes industry to task, our regulators and legislators cannot be trusted to usher Americans toward better health. In the meantime, it is up to you to take control of your health, and do what is right for you, to live a healthier, longer, drug- and disease-free life. Proper nutrition, exercise, and avoidance of toxins are three critical factors to address in this process, and this e-book contains many helpful tips and information to help you do just that.

By buying organic, you will dramatically reduce your exposure to pesticides, hormones and antibiotics, as those are used on nearly all GE crops. When shopping locally, know your local farmers. Many are too small to afford official certification, but many still adhere to organic, sustainable practices. The only way to determine how your food is raised is to check them out, meeting the farmer face to face if possible. Yes, it does take time but is worth it if you are really concerned about your family's health.

Chapter 8:

The Importance of Exercise for Gout

Sufferers

In today's time we are not all farmers and that is part of the problem, we don't have much activity in our daily work. Most of us sit on a chair for 8 hours and the body part that gets the most exercise is our fingers! Not to mention straining our eyes staring in that computer screen all day!

Exercise, where you raise your pulse rate, you burn 100 calories roughly by walking 1 mile. I recommend you walk at a speed that gets you out of breath by walking rapidly. Our overall death rate goes down by 50% through regular exercise. It'll help you carry more oxygen into your cells and it will make major organs of the body work more efficiently—your heart, brain and your thought process will be improved. Your risk of dying from coronary heart disease will drop by 60%!!! "I heard that many people die from exercise" you may ask. It is true that 2% of coronary heart deaths occur during exercise in the form of a heart attack. But don't let this deter you; you have to put it in perspective. Fifty percent of the people who die from heart disease, from that blood clot that closes off that vessel, are caused while they are sleeping! Are you going to quit sleeping because of the fact that 50% of people die from heart failure during their sleep? You see there is no indictment against exercise! Why does this happen while you are sleeping, doesn't your heart rest? Yes it's true but the mechanism is strange. If you eat a fatty meal topped off with ice cream for dessert, and then go to bed even after 3 hours, as you rest your circulation decreases and the heart slows. You already have a coronary artery that's almost closed off—85% of the lumen is closed and the red cells are sticky, they usually travel through that little hole, one at a time but now 5 of them are clogging, getting stuck together, they simply can't get through because they are sticky and have fat on them. The efficiency in carrying oxygen is cut down by 1/3, so you are only getting 2/3 of the oxygen, if it gets through. The sludging of the cells, the plates also become sticky and that causes a blood clot to develop which closes the hole and no blood gets through at all. If it's a small vessel you have a minor heart attack, if it's a large vessel you have a major heart attack and if the left main coronary arteries are included, 40% of the people die immediately!

So how much exercise should you do? A study of 20 college students who were very athletic and were either part of the football team, basketball team and so on, were hired during the summer months to lie flat in bed at the college for 3 weeks straight. They were fed in bed and even had bedpans for them not to go to the bathroom. Pretty extreme eh? At the end of the 3 week period they discovered that these healthy boys deteriorated physiologically the equivalent of 30 years of aging. Hopefully, they were able to return these people to normal health very rapidly with proper exercise and some physiotherapy. When these boys got out of bed, they weren't even able to stand up, they needed help! So this should motivate you, when you wake up in the morning to jump out of bed and go for a walk or even walk the dog, put in wood, whatever it is, do something.

Realize that you will age very rapidly if you do not exercise every day. How much exercise do I do and how do I know when to stop? While walking fast for about 30 minutes, your target pulse should be 170 minus your age and the maximum should be 220 minus your age. This is the general rule of course, there are some exceptions with people that have special problems so check with your doctor and let him monitor your pulse. Don't get it over 220 minus you are because you will get into trouble and risks being part of the 2% that die of a heart attack while exercising! The idea is to walk about 3 miles a day, 6 days a week and you will burn up to 1800 kilocalories. Walk at least 10 miles a day if you want it to be most effective and beneficial to your health. On average, walking a 10 miles may take roughly 150 minutes when going along at a natural or brisk pace. Trail and uphill walking will also take longer to complete a mile, but ultimately will burn more calories. How tall you are needs to be taken in consideration, since stride length is reduced in shorter people, making it harder to walk at higher speeds. Moreover, your weight will also determine how many total calories will be burned. When looking at how much weight is being lost when walking 10 miles, the actual weight of the person is crucial to determine the amount of calories burned as well as the pace. For an average man of 5 feet 8 inches weighing 75 kg, the approximate number of calories burned during a brisk walk at 4 miles per hour would be 800 to 900 calories if the course was relatively flat, taking him two hours and a half to complete. If you have time to walk

10 miles daily, this amount is probably more than enough for anyone to lose weight, especially if nutritious dietary changes also are made (*source: www.livestrong.com*)

In the context of different foods, by eating a hot fudge sundae, you'll need to walk 4.5 miles to burn it up. A Big Mac? You'll need to walk 7 miles to burn it off. Lose 5 pounds? To lose 1 pound of fat is the equivalent of 40 miles walking, running or crawling, you pick! So it's not worth it beloved, you really got to work hard if you want to burn that fat from your body. Why go to such extremes, watch your diet and if you eat a high carb diet by limiting your fat and protein intake by 10% each, you will lose the weight!

When you exercise, it energizes the whole body! You might say, "Well I'm too old now to start exercising or to begin eating properly." We have found with atherosclerosis, that it totally disappears in 2 years if you don't eat any fat and it doesn't make a difference how old you are when you start. You don't have to be sick to get better, you don't inherit disease from your family genes, you inherit bad habits from your family! The beta endorphins go up when you exercise, they rev the body up, our body works more efficiently, we fight disease better and causes us to be a happy people. Exercise is the natural opiate which gives you a natural high! It will increase the speed at which you heal from injury, it will decrease the pain you might suffer, it will increase your pleasurable feelings, it will improve your blood circulation and it will provide better oxygen supply to all the vital organs making you a more efficient human being. It will lower uric acid levels that in turn will lessen your gout attacks. Exercise tones your heart muscle and heart rhythm. Exercise decreases depression, it decreases your appetite, it increases your fitness, it increases your reflexes and you will look and feel better! It helps diabetes, it helps your glucose tolerance, it avoids calcium leaving your system and it prevents osteoporosis. Osteoporosis is a disease characterized by low bone mass and deterioration of bone tissue. This leads to increased bone fragility and risk of fracture (broken bones), particularly of the hip, spine, wrist and shoulder. Osteoporosis is often known as "the silent thief" because bone loss occurs without symptoms. Osteoporosis is sometimes confused with osteoarthritis, because the names are similar. Osteoporosis is a bone disease; osteoarthritis is a disease of the joints and surrounding tissue. Fractures from osteoporosis are more common than heart attack, stroke and breast cancer combined. At least one in three women and one in five men will suffer from an osteoporotic fracture during their lifetime. If you like aerobics, research has proven that this form of exercise really works more than others due to the fact that it stresses your lungs and your heart becoming more efficient, increasing endurance and the muscle efficiency increases that you don't feel tired. You feel ready to go up at any time because the energy available is instantly stored up in the muscle and in the liver in large quantities. Furthermore, long distance running burns fat more efficiently. Exercise causes you to become a more optimistic, enthusiastic and creative person. You will find that if you exercise regularly that you do not tire out because you increase that capacity to store energy.

Caffeine causes tremendous energy to be released in the form of fat. It is true should we use this before long endurance exercises, it will cause us some problems due to being a diuretic and causes us to lose water. Water is the most important thing when you exercise. It's essential for proper circulation, for urine production and temperature control. If you lose as much as 3% of your body weight in water, it begins to interfere with the efficiency, in whatever sport you are involved in or whatever labour you are involved in. Lose 10% of your body weight by water and you will go into a heat stroke! Gout sufferers should always be well hydrated due to the risk of getting a flare-up if you are dehydrated for a long period of time.

So what do you then? If you are going to exercise or play a sport, drink 24 ounces of water 2 hours before and then about 14 ounces just a few minutes before you exercise or compete. Then try and drink 7 ounces every 15 minutes while exercising or competing. What about drinking Gatorade to replace the potassium you lose while exercising? Not needed, eating one banana after exercising provides you with 7 times more potassium than 10 ounces of Gatorade or any other advertised products out there. Any fruit you eat after exercise will help replenish your carbohydrates, potassium and other minerals you lost while exercising. Water is the most important thing to take a lot of while exercising or playing a sport.

Finally, exercise will also banish fatigue, assure you of energy and will lower your risk of developing a degenerative disease. It's never going to occur one day whereby you will have a magic pill, powder, liquid, capsule to take and eat all the fat you like and not expect to get a disease. And it doesn't really matter what type of exercise you do, as long as you do some type of activity that raises your heart rate, it can be walking, jogging, running, aerobics, tennis, basketball, hockey, swimming, dancing, boxing, martial arts, weight-lifting, even working around the house and doing the little things during a day that make a big difference towards your health. Take the stairs instead of the elevator, walk to the 7 Eleven to get your milk instead of driving there for a block, run up the stairs of your house instead of walking them slowly. Shovel your driveway instead of hiring a snow removal company to do it for you. I gave you some ideas, now it is time to take action! Let's go, get out and do a physical activity!

In conclusion, I hope you take all this knowledge and take immediate action, not starting tomorrow or after-tomorrow...Today!!! Take this diet and begin it today, there are no excuses since you have over 100 recipes to get started with and which some of them take barely any time to prepare and cook. You need to change your ways or else face your health worsening causing you more pain and heartache, more bills for prescription drugs, the risk of depression and even death! Remember before you begin this diet to take a blood test and record your uric acid level and after even 30 days, 45 days or 60 days of following this e-book's gout diet plan, remember to take another blood test and record your uric acid level. If your uric acid levels haven't decreased significantly then just request for a full refund on the price you paid for this e-book and you will get fully refunded on your credit card immediately with no questions asked. I'm not here to play games and just write an e-book for the hell of it and waste your time. Others on the web will sell you lies about all you have to do to cure gout is take this or that and you'll be cured! They make it look and sound so easy. The truth is it ain't! You need to be disciplined into sticking with my gout diet plan or else forget it. Go back to your old eating habits and good luck to you. I wrote this e-book because too many gout sufferers were writing to me how they were on a potato diet, eating nothing but potatoes all day, or they were drinking nothing but alkaline water to cure their gout, another funny one was just juicing vegetables 3 times a day, so I knew I had to do something to educate gout sufferers around the world.

For those who will go through with the gout diet plan, I encourage you to write to me with some feedback on your experience. I love to hear positive changes in peoples lives, it makes me happy! Some people, no matter how much they control their diet, have more of a problem with reoccurring flare-ups than others. That is the truth and that is the reason that I can't make the claim that your gout can be cured. I'd be just another liar or snake oil salesman trying to make a buck off of you but it doesn't mean that nobody out there hasn't cured their gout because I do believe in the body's ability to heal. There are examples of people out there but not too many. The truth is for many of yous, attempting to cure your gout will cause you more serious health issues that I've described earlier in the e-book. All I am saying is, if you do want to attempt it, please make sure that you talk to your doctor beforehand so he can monitor the progression. Thank you for reading my e-book **Gout and You: The Ultimate Gout Diet and Cookbook**. What are you waiting for? Get started today!

PURINE INDEX

Here is a sample list of Purine Rich Foods you definitely want to avoid and if you do like some of these foods make sure to limit them as much as possible.

		(More than 80 mg / dl – more purine further)
Uric acid in mg/100gr	Purines in mg/100gr	food
3360 – 3600	1400 – 1500	Meat extract
1200 – 1476	500 – 615	Sweetbreads
802	335	Sprat
684	285	Yeast
600	250	Porcine
552	230	Beef liver
480	200	Sardines

360	150	Mackerel with skin
345	144	Trout
336	140	Sardine
288	120	Calf liver
276	115	Pork shoulder with skin
254	106	Tuna
254	106	Goose meat
211,2	88	Pork cutlet
204	85	Ham

Relatively Low Purine Meat and Fish Product (20 – 80 mg / dl, approximately)

Uric Acid in mg/100gr	Purines in mg/100gr	Food
58	24	Pudding
60	25	Crab
62	26	Sausage
80	33	Smoked

91	38	Beef brisket
96	40	Bratwurst
96	40	Plaice
96	40	Pork belly
108	45	Rabbit
108	45	Chicken legs
108	45	Cod
110	46	Roast pork
120	50	Pork chop
153,6	64	Beef(fillet)
158	66	Mackerel without skin
158	66	Beef tongue
170,4	71	Peas (cooked)

Low purine foods are mainly found in plant foods as in carbohydrates like I've been telling you over and over in this e-book and also in most dairy products but in low fat dairy products. Here are some example with low purine content:

Uric Acidin mg/100gr	Purinesin mg/100gr	Low PurineDiet
		Food
0	0	Milk
0	0	Yogurt
0	0	Quark
4,8	2	Egg
7,2	3	Cucumber
10	4	Hard cheese
9,6	4	Griess
9,6	4	Potatoes
9,6	4	Lettuce
9,6	4	Radish
9,6	4	Tomatoes
9,6	4	Onion
38	16	Whole Wheat flour

31	13	Camembert

Refer to this link which has an exhaustive list of foods with their purine content →
http://www.acumedico.com/purine.htm

As you see my Gout Diet Plan makes common sense, if you want to lower your uric acid levels, you need to eat 80% of your daily calories as carbohydrates in fresh fruits, vegetables, whole wheat breads, whole wheat pastas, basmati rice, jasmine rice, brown rice. 10% of your daily calories as protein in lean meats, chicken, fish (which is your best source of protein), and beans. 10% of your daily calories in fat as in low fat milk, yogurt, eggs, cheese, butter, nuts. This is so simple that a child can understand and will provide you with the results you need to remain free from more gout attacks and high uric acid levels.

1. AZTEC COUSCOUS

Here you got a tasty vegetarian dish with a Latin flair which will take you 15 minutes of prep time and just 10 minutes to cook it!

Ingredients:

1 cup couscous

1/2 teaspoon ground cumin

1 teaspoon of sea salt or to taste

1 to 1-1/4 cups water

1-3/4 cups black beans or 1 (15-ounce) can

1 cup corn kernels

1/2 cup red onion, finely chopped

1/4 cup fresh cilantro, minced

1 jalapeno, minced

3 Tablespoons roasted garlic olive oil

3 to 4 Tablespoons freshly squeezed lime juice

✳ How to prepare:

- ❖ Place couscous, cumin, and salt in a large heatproof bowl or storage container and pour 1 cup boiling water on top.
- ❖ Cover tightly and let sit until all the liquid is absorbed, about 10 minutes. If the couscous is not quite tender, add an additional 1/4 cup of boiling water, cover, and let sit for a few minutes longer. Fluff up with a fork.
- ❖ Add in the black beans, corn, red onion, cilantro, and jalapeno.
- ❖ Mix in the olive oil and enough lime juice to give the salad a lemony edge.
- ❖ Serve warm or at room temperature.

2. BABY ARTICHOKES SAUTEED WITH VEGGIES

In this tasty vegetarian dish, the baby artichokes are sautéed with carrots, leeks, garlic and wine. You then top it with mild cheese and olives. This dish is served at room temperature which takes 20 minutes of prep time and 35 minutes to cook.

Ingredients:

18 baby artichokes
1/2 cup olive oil
3 large carrots, peeled and cut into small dice
3 leeks (white part and 3 inches green), well rinsed, dried, and chopped
4 cloves garlic, minced
Salt and freshly ground black pepper, to taste
1/2 cup dry white wine
1 Tablespoon fresh lemon juice
4 ounces Montrachet or other soft mild chevre
Garnish with some olives

✻ How to prepare:

- ❖ Cut the stem and 1/4 inch of the top from each artichoke.
- ❖ Trim the tough outer leaves with a scissor.
- ❖ Heat the oil in a saucepan large enough to hold all the artichokes upright over medium-high heat.
- ❖ Add the carrots, leeks, and garlic.
- ❖ Sauté, stirring frequently, for 10 minutes.
- ❖ Season to taste with salt and lots of black pepper.
- ❖ Place the artichokes upright on the bed of vegetables and pour in the wine.
- ❖ Sprinkle the lemon juice over the tops of the artichokes.
- ❖ Cover the pan and simmer over medium low heat for 20 to 25 minutes.
- ❖ Remove from heat and cool to room temperature.
- ❖ Remove the artichokes from the vegetables and set aside.
- ❖ Crumble the chevre cheese into the vegetable mixture and fold gently together.

- ❖ Spoon the vegetable mixture onto a platter or 6 individual serving plates.
- ❖ Arrange the artichokes on top of the vegetables, spooning a few vegetables over the tops.
- ❖ If you are serving on plates, allow 3 artichokes per serving.
- ❖ Garnish with olives and serve at room temperature.

3. BAKED PASTA WITH ZUCCHINI AND MOZZARELLA

Very simple casserole of baked pasta tossed with zucchini, tomatoes, black olives and mozzarella cheese.

Ingredients:

3/4 pound of 100% whole wheat pasta (fusilli, orecchiette or conchiglie)
5 small zucchini cut into 1/2-inch slices
Salt and pepper
1 (28 ounces) can Italian plum tomatoes, drained and chopped
8 black olives, sliced
3 Tablespoons Parmesan cheese, freshly grated
1 teaspoon fresh rosemary sprigs
1/2 pound Mozzarella cheese, cut in 1/2-inch cubes

✳ How to prepare:

- ❖ Cook pasta in boiling salted water.
- ❖ In a large frying pan, heat oil and saute zucchini until lightly browned, about 5 minutes.
- ❖ Season with salt and pepper and transfer to an oiled shallow casserole dish.
- ❖ Preheat oven to 350 degrees F.
- ❖ When pasta is almost cooked, drain and add to zucchini.
- ❖ Add tomatoes, olives, Parmesan, rosemary, and 1/2 of the mozzarella.
- ❖ Sprinkle with a little more salt and pepper if desired and gently mix together.
- ❖ Cover with the remaining mozzarella and bake until cheese is melted and the top slightly browned, about 15 minutes.

4. PESTO WITH BASIL AND SUNFLOWER SEEDS

Quick meal to prepare with pasta that includes basil, garlic, sunflower seeds, parmesan cheese blended with pesto sauce which is prepared in as little as 10 minutes!

Ingredients:

4 cups coarsely chopped fresh basil leaves

1 cup hulled raw sunflower seeds

1/2 cup olive oil

1 cup freshly grated Parmesan

2 Tablespoons sweet butter, at room temperature

2 cloves garlic, crushed

✳ How to prepare:

- ❖ Cook 1 pound of pasta in salted water.
- ❖ When pasta is cooked al dente, combine 3/4 cup pesto with 2/3 cup hot pasta water in a large bowl.
- ❖ Drain pasta and add to the bowl. Toss to combine.
- ❖ Add lemon juice, salt, and pepper to taste. Toss again and serve immediately.
- ❖ Place basil, sunflower seeds, olive oil, Parmesan, butter, and garlic in the bowl of a food processor fitted with the metal blade.
- ❖ Process to a puree, scraping down sides often.
- ❖ Transfer pesto to a small bowl with a lid.
- ❖ Press a sheet of plastic wrap to the surface of the pesto sauce, then seal with the lid. May be refrigerated up to 2 weeks.

5. BEEF TENDERLOIN STUFFED WITH PEPPERS, SPINACH, AND GOAT CHEESE WITH WINE SAUCE

A meal that you can enjoy once a week, I usually have my beef meal on the weekend, although there are many ingredients, prep time will take 15 minutes and cook time is about 50 minutes for a total of 1 hour and 5 minutes, not a difficult recipe.

Ingredients:

1 (3 to 4-pound) organic beef tenderloin, center cut
1 (10-ounce) package frozen chopped spinach, thawed
8 ounces goat cheese, room temperature
1 tablespoon chopped fresh rosemary
1 tablespoon chopped fresh thyme
1 (12-ounce) jar roasted red peppers, drained
Salt and freshly ground pepper
1 bunch fresh basil leaves
2 tablespoons olive oil
2 shallots, minced
1/2 cup port wine
1 cup beef stock
1 tablespoon cornstarch dissolved in 1/4 cup beef stock
1/3 cup tomato paste
1 teaspoon fresh rosemary
1/4 cup more beef stock
2 tablespoons butter, cold, cut into pieces

✳ How to prepare:

- ❖ Butterfly the beef tenderloin by cutting the beef lengthwise down the center about two-thirds of the way through the beef.
- ❖ Open the beef tenderloin. Use a meat mallet to pound the meat to 3/4-inch thickness.

- ❖ Place the spinach in a colander and squeeze out as much of the moisture as possible.
- ❖ Mix together the spinach, goat cheese, fresh rosemary, and thyme in a large bowl.
- ❖ To stuff and roll the beef tenderloin, season the flattened beef with salt and freshly ground pepper.
- ❖ Place the red peppers on top of the beef leaving a 1-inch border.
- ❖ Place the fresh basil leaves on top of the red peppers.
- ❖ Spread the cheese mixture on one end of the peppers and basil. The cheese will be at the center of the rolled beef.
- ❖ Roll the beef around the cheese end in a tight cylinder.
- ❖ Continue rolling jelly roll fashion.
- ❖ Use butcher string or bamboo skewers to secure beef roll.
- ❖ Refrigerate for at least one hour or until ready to serve.
- ❖ Preheat the oven to 375 degrees F.
- ❖ Heat 2 tablespoons olive oil in a large roasting pan over medium high heat.
- ❖ Add the beef tenderloin roll to the pan and quickly brown on all sides.
- ❖ Place the tenderloin on a rack in a roasting pan.
- ❖ Roast for 30 to 40 minutes.
- ❖ Use a meat thermometer to determine doneness.
- ❖ Cook the shallots over medium high heat in the pan used to brown the beef. Cook until just soft.
- ❖ Add the port wine to the pan and cook until the liquid is reduced by half.
- ❖ Add 1 cup beef stock and bring to a boil.
- ❖ Add the dissolved cornstarch and stir until thickened.
- ❖ Add the tomato paste and fresh rosemary.
- ❖ Season with salt and pepper.
- ❖ Remove the stuffed beef tenderloin from the pan and allow to rest for at least 10 minutes.
- ❖ Remove the rack from the roasting pan.
- ❖ Place the roasting pan over medium high heat.
- ❖ Add 1/4 cup of beef stock to the roasting pan to deglaze.
- ❖ Stir to loosen the brown bits from the bottom of the pan.
- ❖ Add the port wine sauce to the roasting pan.
- ❖ Simmer for 2 minutes. Reduce the heat.
- ❖ Stir in the cold butter until just combined.
- ❖ Cut the stuffed beef tenderloin into 1-inch slices.
- ❖ Pour the port wine sauce onto a dinner plate.
- ❖ Place a slice of beef tenderloin on top of the sauce.
- ❖ Garnish with fresh basil leaves.

6. BLACK WALNUT PESTO

Another simple pasta dish that includes walnuts, pine nuts and herbs that makes a delicious pesto sauce. This sauce can also be used as a dip. Prep time for this dish is 15 minutes and cook time of 40 minutes for a grand total of 55 minutes of your time.

Ingredients:

1 head elephant garlic
1 cup olive oil, plus about 2 Tablespoons for basting
1/2 cup fresh basil leaves
1/4 cup fresh cilantro or parsley leaves
1 cup walnuts
1 cup pine nuts
1/2 cup black walnuts
1/4 cup dark-colored miso
1/4 cup lecithin granules

✴ How to prepare:

- ❖ Preheat the oven to 375 degrees F.
- ❖ In a covered, oiled casserole dish, bake the garlic for 40 minutes, basting occasionally with the 2 tablespoons of olive oil.
- ❖ Let cool and then peel.
- ❖ Meanwhile, in a food processor or by hand, chop the basil and cilantro or parsley.
- ❖ Add the garlic and process or chop again.
- ❖ Add the walnuts and pine nuts.
- ❖ Process or chop until finely chopped.
- ❖ Add the miso, lecithin, and remaining cup of olive oil and process until well mixed.
- ❖ Black Walnut Pesto will keep, tightly covered, in the refrigerator for up to 3 weeks, covered with a thin layer of olive oil.
- ❖ Serve it on whole wheat pasta, as a dip, or as a spread for crackers or bread.

7. BRAISED ARTICHOKES WITH TOMATOES AND THYME

Artichokes are sauteed with onions, garlic, thyme, and tomatoes, then served over pasta and sprinkled with Parmesan. The only time-consuming part is trimming down the artichokes. The rest of the preparation is quite easy clocking in at 30 minutes and cook time of 45 minutes for a grand total of 1 hour and 15 minutes.

Ingredients:

1 lemon
4 medium artichokes (about 2 pounds)
1/4 cup olive oil
1 medium onion, minced
4 medium cloves garlic, minced
1 Tablespoon minced fresh thyme leaves
1 teaspoon of sea salt
1/4 teaspoon freshly ground black pepper
1 (28-ounce) can whole tomatoes packed in juice
1 pound whole wheat linguine or long, thin pasta
Freshly grated Parmesan cheese to taste

✳ How to prepare:

- ❖ Cut the lemon in half and squeeze the juice into a large bowl of cold water.
- ❖ Add the lemon halves to the bowl.
- ❖ Work with just one artichoke at a time and dip it into the water bath if it starts to discolor as you proceed.
- ❖ To begin actual preparation, bend back and snap off the tough outer leaves on the artichoke.
- ❖ Remove several layers until you reach leaves that are mostly pale green or yellow except for the tips.
- ❖ Cut off the pointed leaf tops that are dark green. (Trim about 1 inch from a medium artichoke.)

- ❖ Trim the base of the stem and use a vegetable peeler to remove the dark green outside layer of skin from the stem.
- ❖ Use a knife or the vegetable peeler to remove any dark green leaf bases that may still encircle the top of the stem.
- ❖ The next step is to quarter the artichoke lengthwise, leaving part of the stem attached to each piece.
- ❖ Beginning at the stem end of each quarter, slide a small, sharp knife under the fuzzy choke and cut toward the leaf tips.
- ❖ Discard the choke. Cut the cleaned artichoke quarters into 1/4-inch-thick wedges.
- ❖ Drop the wedges into the bowl with the acidulated water. Once one artichoke has been completely trimmed, repeat the procedure with the next artichoke.
- ❖ Heat the olive oil in a large saute pan with a cover.
- ❖ Add the onion and saute over medium heat until translucent, about 5 minutes.
- ❖ Stir in the garlic and saute for 1 minute.
- ❖ Drain the artichokes and add them to the pan along with the thyme, salt, pepper, and 1 cup water.
- ❖ Simmer briskly until most of the water in the pan has evaporated, about 10 minutes.
- ❖ Coarsely chop the tomatoes and add them to the pan along with all of their packing juice.
- ❖ Cover the pan and simmer gently, occasionally using a spoon to break apart the tomatoes, until the sauce thickens and the artichokes soften completely, about 35 minutes.
- ❖ Taste for salt and pepper and adjust seasonings if necessary.
- ❖ While preparing the sauce, bring 4 quarts of salted water to a boil in a large pot.
- ❖ Cook and drain the pasta.
- ❖ Toss the hot pasta with the artichoke sauce.
- ❖ Mix well and transfer portions to warm pasta bowls.
- ❖ Serve immediately with grated Parmesan cheese passed separately.

8. CARAMELIZED LEEKS OVER NOODLES

You don't have to be vegetarian to enjoy the rich flavour of caramelized leeks. This quick and simple dish is amazingly full of flavour and only takes 10 minutes of prep time and 30 minutes of cook time for a total of 40 minutes of your time.

Ingredients:

2 medium leeks
1/2 Tbsp olive oil
1 Tbsp soya margarine
1/2 Tbsp dark brown soft sugar
5 ounces (150 g) noodles
2 heaping Tbsp chopped fresh parsley
1 tsp extra-virgin olive oil

✳ How to prepare:

- ❖ Salt and black pepper to taste.
- ❖ Split the leeks lengthways and wash each layer thoroughly.
- ❖ Slice across into thin strips, including the green part.
- ❖ Heat the olive oil and margarine together over a gentle heat. When the margarine has melted, add the leeks and toss well.
- ❖ Cook slowly, uncovered, for about 10 minutes or until the leeks start to soften.
- ❖ Sprinkle over the sugar. After a couple more minutes, mix well.
- ❖ Continue to cook for 15 to 30 minutes, until the leeks have begun to collapse into a sticky mass.
- ❖ Add small amounts of hot water if required to stop sticking.
- ❖ While the leeks are cooking, cook and drain the noodles.
- ❖ When the leeks are done, add the parsley, olive oil, cooked noodles and seasoning to taste.
- ❖ Toss well and serve.

9. CHICKEN BREASTS ROASTED WITH HONEY, PINE NUTS AND THYME

Honey, thyme, and pine nuts make chicken breasts shine in this dish. The breasts are browned in a heavy skillet and finished in the oven for a moist and flavorful result. Take care not to overcook the chicken or it will become dry and chewy. Your prep time for this dish is only 15 minutes and only 30 minutes to cook it for a total of 45 minutes of your time. This dish makes 6 servings.

Ingredients:

3 Tablespoons honey
4-1/2 Tablespoons olive oil
2 Tablespoons freshly squeezed lemon juice
3/4 teaspoon Worcestershire sauce
3/4 teaspoon dried thyme
3/4 dried oregano
1/4 teaspoon ground mace
4-1/2 Tablespoons pine nuts, somewhat finely chopped
Salt and freshly ground pepper
6 split grain-fed chicken breasts on the bone, each about 3/4 pound (4-1/2 pounds total), excess skin trimmed
1/2 cup dry vermouth or dry white wine

✳ How to prepare:

- ❖ Preheat the oven to 400 degrees with the rack in the center and a heavy roasting pan large enough to hold all the chicken pieces with plenty of room around each piece.
- ❖ Mix the honey, 3-1/2 tablespoons of the olive oil, the lemon juice, Worcestershire sauce, thyme, oregano, and mace in a medium bowl until smoothly combined.
- ❖ Stir in the pine nuts, season with salt and pepper, to taste.
- ❖ Dry the chicken breasts with paper towels and season them generously with salt and pepper.

- ❖ Set a large, heavy skillet over medium-high heat with the remaining 1 tablespoon olive oil.
- ❖ When it's hot, brown the breasts in batches, skin side down, adding more oil if needed, until they are golden and the fat from the skin is rendered, 3 to 5 minutes per batch.
- ❖ When all the breasts are browned, transfer them to the roasting pan, skin side up, and coat each with the honey mixture, spreading it with the back of a spoon (some will drip in the pan).
- ❖ Pour the vermouth around the breasts and place the pan in the oven.
- ❖ Roast until the chicken is just cooked through, 15 to 18 minutes (to check, make a cut in the thickest part of one breast to see if it's white in the center).
- ❖ If at any time the juices threaten to evaporate and burn, add a little more wine or water.
- ❖ Transfer the chicken to a warm platter or plates and reserve the roasting pan.
- ❖ Set the pan directly over low heat (or transfer the juices to a small saucepan) and cook the juices down with any accumulated platter juices, stirring, until it becomes a flavorful, light syrup.
- ❖ Season with more salt and pepper if you like, spoon the juices over the breasts, and serve hot.

10.   CHICKEN CACCIATORE

An Italian favorite, this version of cacciatore uses a quick homemade marinara sauce, mushrooms, garlic, and olives for a hearty chicken dish. Prep time of 15 minutes and cook time of 1 hour and 30 minutes for a grand total of 1 hour and 45 minutes to make this tasty dish. This recipe shall provide you with 4 servings.

Ingredients:

Marinara Sauce:

1/4 cup olive oil
8 cloves garlic, chopped
1 teaspoon chopped fresh parsley
2 Tablespoons chopped fresh basil
1/2 teaspoon crushed red pepper flakes
2 (28-ounce) cans whole Italian tomatoes

Chicken:

1 whole 3- to 4-pound grain-fed chicken
Salt and black pepper to taste
1/4 cup olive oil (do not use extra-virgin olive oil)
1 medium onion, thinly sliced
3 cloves garlic, sliced
1/3 cup dry sherry
2 to 4 cups Marinara Sauce from above
1/2 to 3/4 pound sliced fresh mushrooms
15 to 20 pitted gaeta olives (substitute kalamata olives if gaeta are unavailable)
4 fresh basil leaves, chopped

✳ How to prepare:

To make sauce:

- ❖ Heat the oil in a large saucepan over medium heat.
- ❖ Add the garlic and cook until soft.
- ❖ Add the parsley, basil, and red pepper flakes and heat to release flavors, about 10 seconds.
- ❖ Drain the liquid from the canned tomatoes and reserve.
- ❖ Crush the tomatoes with your hands and add to the garlic mixture.
- ❖ Add the reserved juice and bring to a simmer.
- ❖ Simmer gently for 30 to 40 minutes, but do not let the sauce reduce or overcook.
- ❖ Refrigerate until needed. Makes 6 cups.

To make chicken:

- ❖ Cut the chicken into 8 pieces and season with salt and pepper.
- ❖ Over medium-high heat, heat the olive oil in a skillet large enough to hold the chicken pieces without crowding.
- ❖ When the oil is hot, carefully add the chicken pieces, being careful as it will splatter.
- ❖ Brown the chicken on both sides and remove from the pan.
- ❖ Add the onion and cook for 1 to 2 minutes, or until soft.
- ❖ Add the garlic and cook for 1 minute more.
- ❖ Drain off the oil and add the chicken back to the pan.
- ❖ Add the sherry and cook over high heat, scraping any browned bits from the bottom of the pan, until reduced by half.
- ❖ Add 2 cups of the Marinara Sauce.
- ❖ Use 4 cups if needing extra sauce for a side dish of pasta. (Freeze any remaining sauce.)
- ❖ Reduce heat and gently simmer for about 30 minutes, turning chicken pieces once or twice.
- ❖ Add the mushrooms, olives, and basil.
- ❖ Continue simmering for 15 minutes more.
- ❖ Turn off heat and let rest for 15 minutes. Skim fat from the surface. Taste and adjust seasoning. Serve hot.

11.   CHICKEN WITH FORTY CLOVES OF GARLIC

Do not fear the large amount of garlic in this recipe. Garlic cloves are nutty and mellow when cooked whole. Once you try it, you may end up adding even more garlic, because they are so delicious. This classic chicken recipe includes vegetables for a meal in one pot. Prep time for this dish is 20 minutes and cook time is 1 hour and 15 minutes, there's also pre-soak time of 15 minutes, so total time is 1 hour and 50 minutes but it does yield 6 servings.

Ingredients:

2 Tablespoons olive oil
1/2 teaspoon dried rosemary leaves, crumbled
1/2 teaspoon dried thyme leaves
1/4 teaspoon crumbled dried sage leaves
2 Tablespoons fresh lemon juice
40 cloves garlic, whole, peeled (about 2 to 3 heads)
3 carrots, cut into 4-inch lengths, large ends halved lengthwise
6 baby new potatoes, scrubbed, skins on
1/2 pound pearl onions, blanched and peeled
1 whole large grain-fed chicken (4 to 4-1/2 pounds)
Sea salt and freshly ground black pepper

✳ How to prepare:

- ❖ Soak top and bottom of 3-1/4-quart (3.25 L) clay cooker in water for 30 minutes; drain.
- ❖ Line bottom and sides of cooker with parchment paper.
- ❖ Combine olive oil, rosemary, thyme, sage, and lemon juice in a large zip-top bag. Squish to combine.
- ❖ Add garlic cloves, carrots, potatoes, and pearl onions.
- ❖ Seal bag and turn until all vegetables are coated.
- ❖ Scoop out the vegetables (reserving the marinade) and place them around the outer edge of the clay cooker, leaving room for the chicken in the center.

- ❖ Use the remaining marinade to coat the chicken, rubbing it into the skin.
- ❖ Place the chicken in the center of the clay cooker, breast-side up.
- ❖ Sprinkle chicken and vegetables generously with salt and pepper. Cover.
- ❖ Place in a cold oven and set temperature to 475 degrees F. (250 degrees C.).
- ❖ Bake until chicken is tender and juices run clear when thigh is pierced, about 1-1/4 hours.
- ❖ Remove cover and bake an additional 5 to 10 minutes until chicken is crisp and brown.
- ❖ Carve chicken and drizzle with pot gravy.
- ❖ Serve with the whole garlic cloves and vegetables.

12.   CHILLED BROCCOLI AND OLIVE SOUP

Leeks, broccoli, and green olives form the basis of this cold, creamy soup. It is perfect for a warm day. Make this the day before so you can chill it overnight. Prep time for this soup is 15 minutes and cook time is 20 minutes for a grand total of 35 minutes. You've got about 4 to 6 servings with this recipe.

Ingredients:

3 cups broccoli florets, rinsed (about 2 pounds fresh broccoli)
1 cup water
2 Tablespoons butter
1 leek (some green top included), rinsed well and sliced
3 cups chicken stock or broth
3/4 cup pimiento-stuffed green olives
Cayenne pepper
1-1/2 cups half-and-half

✱ How to prepare:

* ❖ Combine broccoli and water in a large saucepan, bring water to the boil, lower heat, cover, and steam for 10 minutes or till tender.
* ❖ In the meantime, heat butter in a small skillet, add leek, and saute for 3 minutes.
* ❖ Combine broccoli, cooking liquid, and leek in a blender or food processor, puree, and pour into a large saucepan.
* ❖ Add chicken stock and stir well.
* ❖ Combine olives, cayenne, and half-and-half in blender or food processor, blend till smooth, add to broccoli mixture, and blend well with a whisk.
* ❖ Chill soup overnight.

13. CLASSIC PESTO

This classic Italian sauce is so easy and versatile; you'll want to keep some always on hand in the refrigerator. Pesto is traditionally made with pine nuts, garlic, olive oil, basil, and Parmesan cheese. It's most popular use is tossed with pasta. Walnuts may be substituted for pine nuts in a pinch. Prep time is only 5 minutes for this sauce and should yield you ¾ of a cup.

Ingredients:

2 tablespoons coarse-chopped walnuts or pine nuts
2 garlic cloves, peeled
3 tablespoons extra-virgin olive oil
4 cups basil leaves (about 4 ounces)
1/2 cup (2 ounces) grated fresh Parmesan cheese
1/4 teaspoon sea salt

✳ How to prepare:

- ❖ You will need a food processor or strong blender. With the motor running, drop the pine nuts and garlic through the feed chute.
- ❖ Process until finely minced.
- ❖ Add the olive oil and pulse three times.
- ❖ Add basil, Parmesan cheese, and salt to the processor bowl.
- ❖ Process until finely minced, scraping down sides.
- ❖ Add to whole wheat pasta of your choice

14. COUSCOUS SALAD WITH DRIED CRANBERRIES AND PECANS

Along with couscous, cranberries, and pecans, this salad also includes peas, scallions, cucumbers, and fresh basil. It is topped with an easy lemon garlic dressing. The salad may be served warm, at room temperature or chilled. Your prep time is 15 minutes and cook time is also 15 minutes for a grand total of 30 minutes. This recipe provides you with 4 servings.

Ingredients:

1 cup shelled pecans
1-1/2 cups couscous
1 cup dried cranberries
1/2 teaspoon turmeric
2 cups boiling water
1 cup thawed frozen peas
3 scallions, very thinly sliced
2 medium cucumbers, peeled, seeded, and diced
1/4 cup shredded fresh basil

Lemon Dressing:

Zest of 1 lemon
1/3 cup lemon juice
3 garlic cloves, minced
1/2 teaspoon salt
Freshly ground black pepper
1/3 cup olive oil

✳ How to prepare:

- ❖ Toast the pecans in a shallow pan in a preheated 350-degree Farenheit oven until very fragrant, about 7 minutes. Set aside to cool.
- ❖ Place the couscous, cranberries, and turmeric in a large bowl.
- ❖ Pour in the boiling water, stir, then cover the bowl with a large plate or foil.
- ❖ Let sit for 10 minutes.
- ❖ Remove the cover, then fluff the couscous with a fork.
- ❖ Cover again and let sit 5 more minutes.
- ❖ Stir in the pecans, peas, scallions, cucumbers, and basil.
- ❖ Combine the dressing ingredients in a jar with a tight-fitting lid and shake vigorously.

15.   PROVENCAL-STYLE COD FISH

This easy Provencal-style cod fish recipe can be on the table within 30 minutes. Prep time is 10 minutes, cook time 20 minutes. Bell peppers, olives, and tomatoes give a burst of flavor to otherwise bland cod fish. Any firm whitefish such as halibut or grouper may be substituted for the cod. You'll get about 4 servings with this recipe.

Ingredients:

1 red, yellow, or green bell pepper (sweet capsicum), cored, seeded, and sliced into 1/2-inch strips
1 medium sweet onion, halved and sliced into 1/2-inch strips
10 whole cloves of garlic, peeled
1 Tablespoon extra-virgin olive oil
2 cups canned crushed tomatoes
12 kalamata olives
1/2 teaspoon Caribbean seasoning blend or lemon pepper
4 (about 5 ounces each) cod fish filets (see Notes)
Sea salt and black pepper to taste, optional

✳ How to prepare:

- ❖ Over medium-low heat, saute bell peppers, onions, and whole garlic cloves in olive oil until vegetables are limp.
- ❖ Add crushed tomatoes, olives, and seasoning or lemon pepper.
- ❖ Continue cooking until garlic cloves are easily pierced with a fork. (Add a bit of water if the mixture becomes too dry.)
- ❖ Raise heat to medium. Add cod filets to the mixture.
- ❖ Saute until cod is cooked through and flakes easily with a fork.
- ❖ Season to taste with sea salt and pepper, if desired.
- ❖ Serve cod filets with the Provencal sauce over the top.

16. COCOA SPICED SALMON

Cocoa, dry mustard, and flavorful spices make an interesting dry rub seasoning mix for barbecued fresh salmon. If you are unable to grill the fish, you may broil it in your oven. Prep time is 10 minutes and cook time is 15 minutes for a grand total of 25 minutes and will provide you with 4 servings.

Ingredients:

2 Tablespoons olive oil
1 Tablespoon brown sugar
1/4 teaspoon dry mustard
Dash of ground cinnamon
1 teaspoon sweet Hungarian paprika
1/2 teaspoon cocoa powder
2 teaspoons chili powder
1/2 teaspoon ground cumin
1/4 teaspoon freshly ground pepper
1-1/2 teaspoons kosher salt
1-1/2 pounds salmon filet (see Notes)

.

Mustard Sauce:

1/4 cup dry mustard
1/4 cup sugar
2 Tablespoons hot water

✳ How to prepare:

- ❖ Heat a grill on medium-high heat.
- ❖ Smear 1 teaspoon of the olive oil over the bottom of a shallow aluminum pan. (Alternatively, you may form a tray out of a double layer of heavy foil. Be sure to place it on a cookie sheet for stability.)

- ❖ Whisk together sugar, dry mustard, cinnamon, paprika, cocoa powder, chili powder, cumin, pepper, and salt.
- ❖ Coat both sides of the salmon filet with remaining olive oil.
- ❖ Place in grill pan skin-side down.
- ❖ Sprinkle generously with the cocoa spice mixture and pat down. You may have some spice mix left over.
- ❖ Store in a glass jar in a cool, dark place up to 6 months.
- ❖ Grill salmon about 10 minutes per inch of thickness, until salmon flakes easily with a fork.
- ❖ Do not overcook or it will become dry.
- ❖ <u>Mustard Sauce:</u>
- ❖ Whisk together dry mustard, sugar, and hot water until smooth.
- ❖ Serve as a condiment with Cocoa Spiced Salmon.

17. GRILLED VEAL CHOPS AND ZUCCHINI WITH ROSEMARY

Boned veal chops are marinated in lemon oil, then skewered on rosemary sprigs and grilled with zucchini. Plan ahead for marination time, 3 hours or overnight. If you cannot use a grill, you can use your oven broiler or a very hot oven. Prep time for this recipe is 3 hours and 15 minutes but cook time only 15 minutes for a total of 3 hours and 30 minutes yielding you about 4 servings.

Ingredients:

4 teaspoons freshly grated lemon zest
1 tablespoon minced fresh rosemary plus four 4-inch woody branches
2 tablespoons fresh lemon juice
1/3 cup olive oil
4 (1-1/4-inch-thick) organic loin veal chops, boned, leaving the tails attached
2-1/2 pounds zucchini, scrubbed and cut diagonally crosswise into 1/3-inch-thick slices

✳ How to prepare:

- ❖ In a large shallow dish stir together 3 teaspoons of the zest, 2-1/2 teaspoons of the minced rosemary, the lemon juice, the olive oil, and salt and pepper to taste until the marinade is combined well.
- ❖ Wrap each tail flush against the loin portion of each veal chop and with a metal skewer pierce a hole through the tail and the loin portion.
- ❖ Sprinkle the tail of each veal chop with 1/4 teaspoon of the remaining zest, 1/8 teaspoon of the remaining minced rosemary, and salt and pepper to taste.
- ❖ Wrap each tail flush against the loin portion, and skewer each veal chop through the pierced holes with a rosemary branch.
- ❖ Add the veal chops to the marinade and let them marinate, covered and chilled, turning them once and adding the zucchini to the marinade for the last hour, for at least 3 hours or overnight.
- ❖ Grill the veal chops on a rack set about 6 inches over glowing coals for 7 minutes on each side for medium-rare meat.
- ❖ Grill the zucchini for 3 minutes on each side, or until it is just tender.

18. LAMB SIRLOIN WITH LENTILS AND GRATIN POTATOES

A simple dish but long on the ingredients list but simple to make and delicious. Prep time clocks in at only 15 minutes while cook time clocks in at 30 minutes for a total of 45 minutes of your precious time. This recipe should yield you 4 servings.

Ingredients:

Lamb:

4 thick organic lamb sirloin steaks or chops (about 7 ounces each)
3 to 4 Tablespoons olive oil
1 sprig fresh thyme
3/4 cup lentils (lentilles de Puy)
1 medium carrot
1/2 small head celeriac
1 medium leek
2 Tablespoons coarsely chopped fresh parsley
1/4 cup vinaigrette dressing
Sea salt and freshly ground black pepper

.

Gratin Potatoes:

1 pound medium, slightly waxy boiling potatoes (Yukon Gold preferably)
1-1/4 cups milk
1-1/4 cups heavy cream
1 clove garlic, sliced
1 sprig fresh thyme
1 bay leaf
3/4 cup grated Gruyére cheese

✳ How to prepare:

- ❖ Remove the central bone from the lamb chops.
- ❖ Trim off fat and neaten into nice "rump" or rounded shapes.
- ❖ Place in a bowl or plastic bag with half of the olive oil and the leaves from the thyme sprig.
- ❖ Set aside to marinate in the fridge.
- ❖ Cook the lentils in boiling salted water for about 15 minutes.
- ❖ Drain and season with salt and pepper.
- ❖ Cut the carrot, celeriac, and leek into 1/2-inch squares (we call this a brunoise).
- ❖ Heat the remaining oil in a saucepan and saute the vegetables until lightly browned, 5 to 7 minutes.
- ❖ Add the lentils and half the parsley, then bind with 2 tablespoons of the vinaigrette.
- ❖ Set aside.
- ❖ For the gratin potatoes, preheat the oven to 400 F (200 C).
- ❖ Peel the potatoes and slice thinly (use a mandoline or the slicing blade of a food processor).
- ❖ Bring the milk and cream to a boil with some sea salt, the garlic, and herbs, and simmer for a couple of minutes.
- ❖ Add the sliced potatoes and simmer for about 5 minutes until just tender.
- ❖ Drain in a colander set over a bowl to catch the creamy milk.
- ❖ Mix the potatoes gently with two-thirds of the gruyere cheese.
- ❖ Layer neatly into four medium ramekins or gratin dishes, seasoning in between the layers with salt and pepper.
- ❖ Spoon a little of the saved creamy milk on top of each ramekin and sprinkle with the last of the cheese.
- ❖ Place the ramekins on a baking sheet and bake for 8 to 10 minutes until the cheese just turns a golden brown.
- ❖ Meanwhile, heat a heavy-bottomed nonstick frying pan until really hot.
- ❖ Remove the lamb steaks from the bowl or plastic bag, wiping off any thyme leaves, and brown for 3 to 5 minutes on each side, seasoning lightly as they cook.
- ❖ The lamb should be served lightly pink -- medium rare.
- ❖ Reheat the lentils and spoon onto the center of four plates.
- ❖ Place the lamb steaks on top (slice them first, if you like).
- ❖ Deglaze the frying pan with the last of the vinaigrette, stirring for a minute, then spoon these juices over the lamb.
- ❖ Sprinkle with the remaining parsley.
- ❖ Serve the gratin potatoes, still in their individual dishes, on the same plate.

19.   LINGUINI WITH PESTO SAUCE

New potatoes and green beans tossed with a basic pesto sauce of basil, garlic, pine nuts, olive oil, and parmigiano cheese is a marriage made in heaven when tossed with whole wheat linguine pasta. Prep time is only 15 minutes as well as coo time for a total of 30 minutes.

Ingredients:

4 ounces (120 gr) small basil leaves
1 garlic clove, chopped
1 ounce (30 gr) pine nuts
1/4 cup (60 cc) extra-virgin olive oil
2 Tablespoons parmigiano reggiano cheese, freshly grated
Salt
1 pound (450 gr) small tender green beans
1 pound (450 gr) new potatoes, peeled and cut into large dices
1 pound (450 gr) whole wheat linguine pasta
4 ounces (115 gr) parmigiano reggiano cheese, freshly grated for topping

✱ How to prepare:

❖ Wash basil leaves and dry them with a towel. If the basil leaves are large, remove the center stems with a sharp knife.
❖ Place the garlic, basil, pine nuts, and one third of the extra-virgin olive oil in a food processor or blender.
❖ Run the blade, and stop occasionally to push the paste down.
❖ Add some more extra-virgin olive oil.
❖ Process the pesto until it is reduced to a fine paste and all the oil has been added.
❖ Stir in the grated parmigiano cheese (see note below for make-ahead instructions) and salt.
❖ Transfer to a non-metallic bowl or jar.
❖ Cover with a drizzle of olive oil and reserve.
❖ In a stockpot, boil the beans and potatoes in salted water, until tender.
❖ Remove the vegetables from the pot; and in the same water, cook the linguini pasta.

❖ Just before the pasta is al dente (firm but not too soft or overcooked) return the vegetables to the pot, and finish cooking.
❖ Drain the pasta and vegetables, transfer to a bowl, top with the pesto sauce and the grated parmigiano cheese.
❖ Toss, and serve immediately.

20. MOUSSAKA

This classic Greek dish which is one of my favorites, includes not only traditional eggplant and lamb, but also potatoes for a hearty casserole. Prep time for this tasty dish is 1 hour and 15 minutes while cook time clocks in at 45 minutes for a grand total of 2 hours of your time but it will yield you approximately 8 to 10 servings.

Ingredients:

2-3 eggplants (about 1 1/2 pounds), sliced lengthwise in 1/4 inch slices
1 1/2 pounds zucchini, sliced lengthwise in 1/4 inch slices
1 1/4 pounds potatoes
2 cups breadcrumbs
4 eggs, separated (reserve yolks for Bechamel)
2 tbsp. olive oil
1 medium onion, diced
2 garlic cloves, minced
1 15 oz. can chickpeas, (Garbanzo) drained, rinsed, and mashed
1 15 oz. can diced tomatoes, with liquid
2 tbsp. tomato paste
1/4 tsp. ground cinnamon
1 tsp. dried oregano
1/2 tsp. ground cumin
1 tsp. sugar
Sea salt and pepper to taste
3/4 cup grated Kefalotyri or Parmesan cheese

Bechamel Sauce:

1/2 cup butter (1 stick)
1/2 cup flour
3 cups milk, warmed
4 egg yolks (reserved from above)
A pinch of ground nutmeg

✳ How to prepare:

Preheat the oven to 400 degrees.

Prepare the vegetables:

- ❖ Place the eggplant and zucchini slices in a colander and salt them liberally.
- ❖ Cover with an inverted plate weighted down by a heavy can or jar.
- ❖ Place the colander in the sink so that excess moisture can be drawn out. They will need to sit for at least 15-20 minutes.
- ❖ Peel the potatoes and boil them whole for about 10 minutes. They should not get too soft, just enough to be tender (parboil).
- ❖ Drain, cool, and slice them in 1/4 inch slices. Set aside.
- ❖ Line a baking sheet with aluminum foil and lightly grease.
- ❖ Add a splash of water to the egg whites and beat lightly with a fork or whisk.
- ❖ Spread breadcrumbs on a flat plate.
- ❖ Rinse the eggplant and zucchini slices and blot excess moisture with paper towels.
- ❖ Set the zucchini aside with the potatoes.
- ❖ Dip the eggplant slices in the beaten egg whites and then dredge them in the breadcrumbs, coating both sides.
- ❖ Place breaded eggplant slices on baking sheet and bake for 1/2 an hour, turning them once during cooking.
- ❖ When eggplant is finished cooking, lower the oven temperature to 350 degrees.

Making the Tomato Sauce:

- ❖ Heat olive oil in a large saute pan.
- ❖ Add onion and saute until translucent, about 5 minutes.
- ❖ Add garlic and cook until fragrant, about 1 minute.
- ❖ Add mashed chickpeas to pan with tomatoes, tomato paste, cinnamon, oregano, cumin, sugar, salt, and pepper.
- ❖ Allow the sauce to simmer uncovered so that excess liquid can be cooked out.

Assembling the Moussaka:

- ❖ Lightly grease a 9 x 13 x 3 inch baking pan.

- ❖ Sprinkle the bottom of the pan with breadcrumbs.
- ❖ Leaving a small space around the edges of the pan, cover the bottom of the pan with a layer of potatoes.
- ❖ Top with a layer of eggplant slices.
- ❖ Add tomato sauce on top of eggplant and sprinkle with grated cheese.
- ❖ Add zucchini slices next. Top with another layer of eggplant slices and sprinkle once again with grated cheese.

Making the Bechamel Sauce:

- ❖ Melt butter over low heat. Using a whisk, add flour to melted butter whisking continuously to make a smooth paste.
- ❖ Allow the flour to cook for a minute but do not allow it to brown.
- ❖ Add warmed milk to mixture in a steady stream, whisking continuously.
- ❖ Simmer over low heat until it thickens a bit but does not boil.
- ❖ Remove from heat, and stir in beaten egg yolks and pinch of nutmeg.
- ❖ Return to heat and stir until sauce thickens, being careful not to scorch it.

Ready for the Oven:

- ❖ Pour the béchamel sauce over the eggplant and be sure to allow sauce to fill the sides and corners of the pan.
- ❖ Smooth the béchamel on top with a knife and sprinkle with remaining grated cheese.
- ❖ Bake in 350 degree oven for 45 minutes or until béchamel sauce is a nice golden brown color.
- ❖ Allow to cool for 15–20 minutes before slicing and serving.

21. MOZZARELLA SOUP WITH VEGETABLES AND BLACK OLIVES

This hearty cheese soup uses lower-fat mozzarella with red onions, carrots, celery, and potatoes, plus black olives and hot sauce for kick. Use the food processor to make quick work of chopping the vegetables. Prep time for this dish is only 20 minutes with a cook time at 35 minutes for a total of 55 minutes to prepare this soup dish providing you with 4 servings.

Ingredients:

3 Tablespoons extra-virgin olive oil (the fruitiest you can find)
1 large red onion, peeled and very coarsely chopped
Half of a 1-pound package peeled baby-cut fresh carrots, very coarsely chopped
2 small celery ribs, very coarsely chopped
1 large baking potato (about 12 ounces), peeled and diced
1 large garlic clove, minced
1 whole bay leaf
One 3-inch sprig fresh rosemary or 1/2 teaspoon dried rosemary, crumbled
One 14-1/2 ounce can chicken broth
One 12-ounce can evaporated milk (use skim, if you like)
1/2 cup fresh whole milk
1/2 teaspoon hot red pepper sauce
Half of an 8-ounce package finely shredded mozzarella cheese
1/3 cup sliced pitted ripe olives
Salt and freshly ground black pepper

✳ How to prepare:

- ❖ Heat oil in large, heavy saucepan over moderate heat 1 minute.
- ❖ Shorten preparation time by using a food processor to chop the vegetables.
- ❖ Add red onions, carrots, celery, potatoes, garlic, bay leaf, and rosemary.
- ❖ Cook, stirring often, 5 minutes.

- ❖ Reduce heat to low, cover, and "sweat" vegetables 10 minutes.
- ❖ Add broth, bring to gently boil, cover, and cook until potato is tender, about 15 minutes.
- ❖ Add evaporated milk, milk, and red pepper sauce and bring to a simmer.
- ❖ Off heat, add mozzarella and stir until smooth.
- ❖ Stir in olives and salt and pepper to taste.
- ❖ Discard bay leaf and rosemary sprig, ladle into heated soup bowls, and serve.

22.   OLIVE, ROSEMARY, AND ONION FOCACCIA

Delicious yeast flatbread is rich with the flavors of rosemary and olives. Plan ahead to allow time for the dough to rise. The dough may be made 8 hours in advance and refrigerated. Prep time is 20 minutes and cook time is 45 minutes for a total of 1 hour and 5 minutes which will yield you 6-8 servings.

Ingredients:

1-1/4-ounce package (2-1/2 teaspoons) active dry yeast
1 teaspoon sugar
4-1/2 to 5 cups whole wheat flour
1-1/4 teaspoons sea salt
3 Tablespoons olive oil
2 teaspoons finely chopped fresh rosemary leaves plus whole rosemary leaves
1/4 cup minced onion
1/2 pound Kalamata, Nicoise, or green Greek olives or a combination, pitted and cut into slivers (about 1 cup)
1-1/2 teaspoons coarse salt, or to taste

✳ How to prepare:

- ❖ In the large bowl of an electric mixer fitted with the dough hook stir together the yeast, the sugar, and 1-3/4 cups lukewarm water and proof the yeast mixture for 5 minutes, or until it is foamy .
- ❖ Stir in 4-1/2 cups of the flour, salt, and 2 tablespoons of the olive oil and knead the dough, scraping down the dough hook occasionally and adding as much of the remaining 1/2 cup flour as necessary to form a soft, slightly sticky dough, for 3 minutes.
- ❖ Transfer the dough to a lightly oiled bowl, turn it to coat it with the oil, and let it rise, covered, in a warm place for 1 hour, or until it is double in bulk.
- ❖ Knead in the chopped rosemary, press the dough with lightly oiled hands into a well-oiled 15-1/2-by 10-1/2-inch jelly-roll pan, and let it rise, covered loosely, for 30 minutes.

❖ The dough may be made 8 hours in advance and kept covered and chilled.
❖ Dimple the dough with your fingertips, making 1/4-inch-deep indentations, brush it with the remaining 1 tablespoon oil, and top it with the onion, the olives, the salt, and the whole rosemary leaves.
❖ Bake the focaccia in the bottom third of a preheated 400 degree F. oven for 35 to 45 minutes, or until it is golden and cooked through.
❖ Transfer the focaccia to a rack, let it cool for 10 minutes, and serve it, cut into squares, warm or at room temperature.

23. PASTA WITH CAPERS, OLIVES AND PINE NUTS

This simple pasta dish is rich with the flavor of capers, black olives, garlic, and pine nuts. This is a fast and easy meal to make or use it as a side dish. Prep time for this simple dish is only 10 minutes and cook time only 15 minutes for a total fo25 minutes of your time. You'll get about 6 portions with this recipe.

Ingredients:

3 Tablespoons butter
3 fluid ounces olive oil
3 cloves garlic, minced
3 ounces pine nuts
15 ounces California black olives, sliced
3 Tablespoons capers, rinsed, minced
1 Tablespoon basil, cut into chiffonade
1 teaspoon oregano, minced
1 teaspoon flat parsley, minced
1 pound of whole wheat pasta, any shape
Salt, to taste
Black pepper, ground, to taste
2 ounces Parmesan cheese, grated

✳ How to prepare:

❖ Combine the butter with the olive oil and heat over medium heat in a large saute pan.
❖ Add the garlic and pine nuts, reduce the heat to low, and continue to cook until the nuts are just beginning to turn golden in color.
❖ Add the olives, capers, basil, oregano, parsley, salt, and pepper.
❖ Toss until the products are incorporated and heated thoroughly.
❖ Cook the pasta in a large saucepan of boiling salted water until al dente.
❖ Drain well.

❖ Toss the drained pasta with the nut-olive mixture over medium heat until the products are incorporated and heated thoroughly.
❖ Season to taste with salt and black pepper.
❖ Sprinkle each portion with grated Parmesan cheese.

24.   PASTA NICOISE SALAD

Pasta salad is loaded with chicken and vegetables, bound with a simple homemade dressing flavored with rosemary. This salad is fresh, bright with flavor, and colorful on the plate. Add some crusty bread, and you have a filling, satisfying meal. For variation, try substituting tuna for the chicken. Prep time for this salad is 20 minutes and only 15 minutes of cook time for a total of 35 minutes yielding 4 servings.

Ingredients:

1 pound pasta (penne, colored corkscrews or bows)
1/4 cup lemon juice
1/4 cup extra virgin olive oil
1/4 cup diced red onion
1 garlic clove, minced
1/4 teaspoon dried rosemary
1/2 pound green beans, halved lengthwise
1-1/2 cups diced cooked (or barbequed) grain-fed chicken
3 plum tomatoes, cut into sixths
2 hard-boiled eggs, cut into eighths
1/4 cup chopped flat-leaf parsley
1 Tablespoon capers, drained
Anchovy fillets and black olives, to taste
Salt and pepper, to taste

✳ How to prepare:

❖ Cook pasta in boiling salted water until just tender.
❖ Drain well and rinse with cold water.
❖ Shake off excess moisture.
❖ Combine lemon juice, oil, red onion, garlic, rosemary, salt, and pepper.
❖ Pour half of dressing over pasta and toss well.
❖ Cook beans until just tender. Drain, rinse with cold water and drain again. Toss beans with half of remaining dressing.
❖ Arrange pasta in serving bowl.

❖ Surround with beans, chicken, tomatoes, and hard-boiled eggs.
❖ Sprinkle remaining dressing over salad.
❖ Top with parsley, capers, anchovies, and black olives.

25. PASTA: SAUTEED SPINACH AND CHICK PEAS WITH LEMON AND THYME

Vegetarian pasta dish with spinach, chick peas, and garlic makes a filling main dish. Plan ahead to soak the chick peas overnight. Prep time is a short 10 minutes, cook time is 55 minutes for a grand total of 1 hour and 5 minutes of your time providing you with 4 portions.

Ingredients:

2/3 cup dried chick-peas (or one 19-ounce can, drained and rinsed thoroughly)

1 bay leaf

1 medium clove garlic, peeled, plus 3 medium cloves, minced

1-1/2 pounds fresh spinach

1/4 cup olive oil

2 teaspoons minced fresh thyme leaves

1 teaspoon sea salt

1 pound farfalle whole wheat pasta

3 Tablespoons lemon juice

✳ How to prepare:

- ❖ Place the chick-peas in a medium bowl and cover them with at least 2 inches of water.
- ❖ Soak overnight and drain.
- ❖ Place the chick-peas, bay leaf, and whole garlic clove in a medium pot and cover them with several inches of water.
- ❖ Bring the water to a boil and simmer gently uncovered until the chick-peas are tender, 35 to 40 minutes.
- ❖ Drain the chick-peas and discard the bay leaf and garlic.
- ❖ Place the chick-peas in a medium bowl and set it aside. (The chick-peas can be covered and refrigerated for up to 2 days.)
- ❖ Bring 4 quarts of salted water to a boil in a large pot for cooking the pasta.

- ❖ Stem the spinach and wash the leaves in a large bowl of cold water, changing the water several times until no sand appears on the bottom of the bowl.
- ❖ Place the spinach with some water still clinging to the leaves in a deep pot or Dutch oven.
- ❖ Cover and set the pot over medium heat.
- ❖ Cook, stirring occasionally, until the spinach has wilted, about 5 minutes.
- ❖ Drain and set aside the spinach.
- ❖ Heat the olive oil in a large skillet.
- ❖ Add the minced garlic and thyme and saute over medium heat for 2 minutes.
- ❖ Add the chick-peas and cook until warmed through, about 1 minute.
- ❖ Add the spinach and salt and heat through, tossing several times, for about 2 minutes.
- ❖ Taste for salt and adjust seasonings if necessary.
- ❖ While preparing the sauce, cook and drain the pasta.
- ❖ Toss the hot pasta with the lemon juice and the spinach sauce.
- ❖ Mix well and transfer portions to warm pasta bowls. Serve immediately.

26. PENNE WITH PEPPERY BROCCOLI AND MOREL SAUCE

Morel mushrooms are sauteed with onions, garlic, and basil to make a delicious sauce for penne pasta and broccoli. Once you soak the mushrooms for 20 minutes, this dish goes together quickly. Prep time and cook time is 20 minutes each for a total of 40 minutes yielding you about 4 to 6 portions.

Ingredients:

1/2 ounce dried morels or similar mushrooms such as cepes or porcini
1/2 cup olive oil
1 onion, minced
1 large garlic clove, minced
1/2 to 1 teaspoon dried hot red pepper flakes, or to taste
1/4 cup minced fresh basil or parsley leaves
1 pound whole wheat penne or similar tubular dried pasta
1 head of broccoli, separated into flowerets and stems peeled and cut into 1-inch pieces (about 1 pound in all)

✱ How to prepare:

- ❖ In a bowl soak the mushrooms in 1 cup boiling water for 20 minutes, drain them, reserving the liquid, and slice them, discarding the tough stems.
- ❖ Strain the liquid through a fine sieve into a bowl and reserve 1/3 cup.
- ❖ In a saucepan heat the olive oil over moderate heat until it is hot, add the onion and the mushrooms, and cook the mixture, stirring, until the onion is pale golden.
- ❖ Add garlic, and the red pepper flakes and cook the mixture, stirring, for 30 seconds.
- ❖ Add the reserved mushroom liquid and salt to taste and simmer the sauce for 1 minute.
- ❖ Stir in the basil.
- ❖ In a large saucepan of boiling salted water cook the penne pasta for 6 minutes, add the broccoli, and cook the mixture for 5 to 6 minutes more, or until the pasta is al dente and the broccoli is just tender.

❖ Drain the mixture, transfer it to a heated bowl, and toss it with the sauce. Serve immediately.

27.   PINE NUT AND SUN-DRIED TOMATO PASTA

Pasta is stir-fried with the rich flavors of pine nuts, sun-dried tomatoes, herbs, and Parmesan for a quick meal. You can have this easy pasta dish on the table in less than 30 minutes. Good as an entree with a salad and bread or use as a side dish. Be sure the pasta is well-drained. The oil will spit and pop when it contacts water. Prep time is only 5 minutes and cook time is only 25 minutes for total time of just half an hour yielding you 4 servings.

Ingredients:

12 ounces whole wheat pasta (fusilli or rigatoni) cooked al dente and drained well
5 Tablespoons olive oil, divided use
2/3 cup toasted pine nuts
2/3 cup oil-packed sun-dried tomatoes, drained and chopped
1/4 cup chopped fresh parsley
1/8 cup chopped fresh basil leaves
1/2 cup grated Parmesan cheese
Sea salt and freshly ground black pepper

✳ How to prepare:

- ❖ Heat a large, heavy skillet over medium-high heat.
- ❖ Add 3 tablespoons of the olive oil and swirl to coat the pan.
- ❖ Add the well-drained pasta and stir-fry until pasta begins to brown at the edges.
- ❖ Remove to a large bowl.
- ❖ To the skillet, add the remaining 2 tablespoons of olive oil.
- ❖ Stir-fry the pine nuts and sun-dried tomatoes for 1 minute.
- ❖ Add to the pasta along with the parsley, basil, and Parmesan cheese.
- ❖ Sprinkle with kosher salt and freshly ground black pepper.
- ❖ Toss to combine and serve immediately.

28. RICOTTA-STUFFED GRAPE LEAVES WITH CAPONATA

Grape leaves are stuffed with ricotta cheese,almonds, and basil, then topped with an easy eggplant caponata sauce. The caponata may be made 1 day in advance. The ingredient list may look daunting, but this is not at all difficult to make. Prep time is 45 minutes and cook time is 2 hours and 30 minutes for a grand total of 3 hours and 15 minutes but does yield you 8 to 10 servings.

Ingredients:

For the Caponata:

2 eggplants (1 pound each), peeled, cut into 1/2-inch slices, then cut into 1/2-inch cubes
Sea salt
1/2 cup olive oil, plus more as needed
2 yellow onions (about 8 ounces each), finely chopped
2/3 cup canned tomato puree
5 Tablespoons red wine vinegar
4 teaspoons sugar
1/4 cup capers, rinsed and drained
3 Tablespoons dried currants, covered with hot water, plumped for 20 minutes, and drained
Salt and freshly ground pepper

For the Grape Leaves:

1 jar (8-ounce) grape leaves in brine
2 cups ricotta cheese, drained well
2 Tablespoons milk
1/2 cup slivered almonds, toasted
1/4 cup chopped fresh basil leaves, plus extra for garnish
Cracked pepper

Olive oil

✻ How to prepare:

To make the caponata:

- ❖ Place the eggplant cubes in a colander, sprinkle with kosher salt, and let stand for about 1 hour.
- ❖ Rinse and pat dry.
- ❖ In a large saute pan, heat the olive oil over medium-high heat.
- ❖ Add the eggplant cubes and saute until very tender and completely cooked through, about 20 minutes.
- ❖ Remove with a slotted spoon and drain on paper towels. Set aside.
- ❖ In the same pan, add 1 to 2 more tablespoons olive oil if needed, and add the chopped onions.
- ❖ Cook over medium heat until the onions begin to soften, about 10 minutes.
- ❖ Add the tomato puree and cook over medium-low heat for 5 minutes.
- ❖ Return the eggplant to the onion-tomato mixture, and add the wine vinegar and sugar.
- ❖ Cook for 5 more minutes.
- ❖ Add the capers and currants, stir well, and cook until the vinegar has cooked of slightly and the ingredients are well blended, about 15 minutes.
- ❖ Add salt and pepper to taste.
- ❖ Set aside, or let cool and then refrigerate overnight.
- ❖ Bring to room temperature before continuing.

To prepare grape leaves:

- ❖ Rinse the grape leaves and pat dry. (This is important because the brine is very salty.)
- ❖ Bring a large pot of water to a boil.
- ❖ Add the grape leaves and boil for 2 minutes.
- ❖ Remove them from the water and place on paper towels to drain. (The grape leaves will probably twist and fold in the boiling process. Don't worry -- they unfold easily.)
- ❖ In a medium bowl, combine the ricotta cheese, milk, almonds, 1/4 cup of the chopped basil, and cracked pepper to taste. Mix well.

To assemble:

- ❖ Preheat the oven to 225 degrees F.
- ❖ Oil a large ovenproof pan or glass baking dish.
- ❖ Place one grape leaf on a work surface with the smooth side down and with the stem side closest to you. The tip of the leaf will be farthest from you.
- ❖ Take 1 tablespoon of the cheese mixture and place it 1/4 inch from the bottom of the grape leaf.
- ❖ Fold the bottom over the cheese mixture.
- ❖ Next, fold in both sides of the grape leaf and roll from the bottom toward the tip.
- ❖ The cheese should be completely encased.
- ❖ Continue with the remaining grape leaves and cheese mixture.
- ❖ Brush the tops of the grape leaves with oil and cover the pan with foil.
- ❖ Set the pan in a larger pan and put them in the oven.
- ❖ Fill the larger pan with hot water to reach halfway up the sides of the baking dish.
- ❖ Bake for 1-1/4 hours.
- ❖ Remove from the oven and let sit, still covered, for 15 minutes.
- ❖ To serve, place three or four stuffed grape leaves on each plate.
- ❖ Drizzle 2 to 3 tablespoons caponata over the grape leaves, and garnish with a little chopped basil.
- ❖ Serve immediately or at room temperature.

29. ROASTED POMEGRANATE CHICKEN

This is a favorite Rosh Hashanah dish of Moroccan Jews. The tangy flavor of pomegranates infuses the sauce for the chicken. Prep time clocks in at 10 minutes and cook time at 50 minutes for a total of 1 whole hour providing you with 4 generous portions.

Ingredients:

1/4 cup olive oil
1 Tablespoon minced garlic
1 (3 1/2 to 4-pound) chicken, quartered
1 pomegranate, halved
1/4 cup dry white wine
Juice of 1 lemon
1 Tablespoon cinnamon
Salt and pepper

✳ How to prepare:

- ❖ Preheat oven to 375 degrees F.
- ❖ In a cup, mix oil and garlic. Brush garlic oil over chicken.
- ❖ Place chicken in a shallow baking dish.
- ❖ Drizzle any remaining oil over chicken.
- ❖ Bake in preheated oven for 45 minutes, basting several times with pan juices, until skin is browned and juices run clear when a thigh is pierced at thickest part with a fork.
- ❖ Remove 1 tablespoon seeds from pomegranates.
- ❖ Set aside for garnish.
- ❖ Squeeze juice form remaining pomegranate through a sieve into a small bowl.
- ❖ In a small nonreactive saucepan, mix pomegranate juice, wine, lemon juice, and cinnamon sugar.
- ❖ Bring to a boil over high heat. Reduce heat to low and cook 5 minutes.
- ❖ Season sauce with salt and pepper to taste.

- ❖ Transfer roasted chicken to a serving platter and pierce each piece several times.

- Pour sauce over chicken.
- Garnish with pomegranate seeds and serve at room temperature.

30. ROASTED VEGETABLES

Roasting carmelizes and brings out the flavor of zucchini, squash, bell peppers, asparagus, and onion. Makes a great side dish or even add between 2 slices of bread, makes a great veggie sandwich. Prep time is only 15 minutes and cook time is 30 minutes for a total of 45 minutes yielding about 4 servings.

Ingredients:

1 medium zucchini, cut into bite-size pieces
1 medium yellow summer squash, cut into bite-size pieces
1 medium red bell pepper, cut into bite-size pieces
1 medium yellow bell pepper, cut into bite-size pieces
1 pound fresh asparagus, cut into bite-size pieces
1 red onion, chopped
3 Tbsp extra virgin olive oil
1 tsp sea salt
1/2 tsp black pepper

✹ How to prepare:

- ❖ Preheat the oven to 450 degrees F.
- ❖ Place the zucchini, squash, bell peppers, asparagus, and red onion in a large roasting pan, and toss with the olive oil, salt, and black pepper.
- ❖ Spread in a single layer.
- ❖ Roast for 30 minutes, stirring occasionally, until the vegetables are lightly browned and tender.

31.   RUSSIAN POTATO SALAD

Beets add the Russian flair to this otherwise traditional potato salad with the addition of carrots and mustard. Make it the day before to let flavors blend, but add the carrots and peas just before serving. Prep time is 15 minutes and cook time is 25 minutes for a total of 40 minutes but will yield you about 10 servings.

Ingredients:

2 pounds white boiling potatoes
1/2 pound beets
1 cup diced carrots
1/2 cup diced celery
1/2 cup minced red onion
1/4 cup sweet pickle relish
1/2 cup chopped Italian parsley
1 cup mayonnaise
1/4 cup white wine vinegar
1/4 cup olive oil
1 Tablespoon Dijon mustard
3/4 teaspoon sea salt
1/8 teaspoon freshly-ground white pepper

✱ How to prepare:

- ❖ Note: This potato salad develops better flavor if it stands overnight, but the potatoes and carrots will become colored by the beets so add them just before serving.
- ❖ Boil the potatoes, beets, and carrots in separate pots until tender.
- ❖ Drain.
- ❖ Peel and dice the potatoes and beets.
- ❖ Place all the vegetables in a large bowl to cool.
- ❖ Add the celery, red onion, pickle relish, and parsley.
- ❖ Mix.
- ❖ Combine the mayonnaise, wine vinegar, olive oil, mustard, salt, and pepper.

❖ Add to the salad and mix gently with a rubber spatula.
❖ Refrigerate the salad for several hours and mix again.
❖ The salad tastes best if prepared the night before serving.

32. SPAGHETTI SQUASH WITH MEDITERRANEAN CHICKEN SAUCE

Spaghetti squash is topped with a rich and creamy sauce made with tomatoes, leeks, garlic, olives, wine, and Parmesan cheese. If you don't like spaghetti squash, serve this incredibly tasty sauce over traditional pasta of your choice. Have all ingredients prepped and ready to go. The spaghetti squash may be cooked in advance and reheated. This goes together pretty fast once you begin. Prep time for this recipe is about 20 minutes and cook time about 1 hour and 25 minutes for total time of 1 hour and 45 minutes and yields you 4 servings.

Ingredients:

1 spaghetti squash
1 leek
4 large garlic cloves, chopped
3 Tablespoons whole wheat flour
1 cup white wine
1-3/4 cups chicken broth (1 can or homemade)
2 large boneless skinless chicken breast halves, cut into 1-inch pieces
1 teaspoon fresh thyme leaves
4 fresh sage leaves, chopped
1 teaspoon kosher salt
Freshly ground black pepper
1 cup heavy cream
2 roma tomatoes, chopped into 1/2-inch dice
1/2 cup black olive wedges
1/2 cup Parmesan cheese
Chopped parsley for garnish

✳ How to prepare:

- ❖ Preheat oven to 375 F.
- ❖ Prick spaghetti squash all over with a skewer.
- ❖ Place spaghetti squash in a pan and bake for 1 hour.
- ❖ When cool enough to handle, cut spaghetti squash in half lengthwise with a serrated knife.
- ❖ Scoop out the seeds, then shred pulp into spaghetti-like strands.
- ❖ Keep warm.
- ❖ Cut leek in half lengthwise and rinse thoroughly in a sink full of water, making sure to remove all dirt.
- ❖ Drain and cut leek into strips about 3 inches long and 1/2 inch wide, including 2 inches of the green part and the center tender leaves.
- ❖ Heat a large, heavy skillet over medium heat. Gently the leeks, stirring often, until leeks begin to brown and caramelize.
- ❖ Add garlic and cook 1 minute.
- ❖ Stir in flour and cook 2 minutes.
- ❖ Carefully pour in wine.
- ❖ Stir and cook 2 minutes, then add chicken broth.
- ❖ Bring to a simmer.
- ❖ Add chicken, thyme, sage, salt, pepper, and cream.
- ❖ Gently simmer until chicken is cooked through and sauce thickens, about 5 to 8 minutes.
- ❖ Add tomatoes, black olives, and Parmesan cheese and cook only until heated through.
- ❖ Serve over cooked spaghetti squash and sprinkle with chopped parsley.

33. SPANAKOPITA

A Greek specialty, these spinach triangle appetizers are made with purchased phyllo sheets and filled with a savory mixture of spinach, cheese, herbs, and spices. Once you get the hang of it, try experimenting with different fillings. I grew up with these at home, one of my favorite greek recipes. Prep time is 45 minutes while cook time is 30 minutes for a total of 1 hour and 15 minutes which will yield you about 40 triangles. Remember this is usually a side dish or snack but can be eaten as alight lunch or supper.

Ingredients:

3 tablespoons olive oil
1 onion, chopped
1/2 cup chopped green onions, greens and whites
3 cloves garlic, minced
2 pounds baby spinach, trimmed, rough chopped
1/2 lemon, juiced
2 eggs, lightly beaten
12 ounces crumbled feta cheese
1 tablespoon coriander seeds, toasted, ground
1/2 teaspoon fresh grated nutmeg
1/2 pound unsalted butter, melted
1 pound phyllo pastry sheets
1/4 cup finely chopped fresh oregano
1/4 cup finely chopped fresh chives
1/2 cup grated Parmesan cheese

✷ How to prepare:

❖ Heat olive oil in a large skillet and place over medium heat.
❖ Saute onions and garlic for 3 minutes until soft.
❖ Add the spinach, season with salt and pepper, and continue to saute until the spinach is limp, about 2 minutes.
❖ Add lemon juice, remove from heat and place in a colander, and squeeze out excess liquid.

- ❖ Set aside to cool.
- ❖ The filling needs to be cool and dry to prevent the phyllo from becoming soggy.
- ❖ In a medium bowl, beat the eggs with feta,coriander, and nutmeg.
- ❖ Season, then fold in the cooled spinach mixture until well blended.
- ❖ Preheat oven to 350 degrees F.
- ❖ Brush 2 baking sheets with some melted butter.
- ❖ Unroll the phyllo dough and lay a sheet flat on a work surface.
- ❖ Take care to keep the phyllo covered with a damp, not wet, towel as you work to prevent drying out and becoming brittle.
- ❖ Brush the sheet with melted butter, then sprinkle evenly with some oregano and chives.
- ❖ Repeat with 2 more sheets of phyllo, stacking on top of each other.
- ❖ With a sharp knife or pizza cutter, cut the sheets lengthwise into thirds to form 2-1/2-inch strips.
- ❖ Do this with all the sheets of dough.
- ❖ Place a heaping teaspoon of filling near 1 corner of the layered phyllo strip.
- ❖ Fold the end at an angle over the filling to form a triangle.
- ❖ Continue to fold the triangle along the strip until you reach the end, like folding up a flag.
- ❖ Brush the top with butter and dust with Parmesan, place on prepared baking sheet, and cover while preparing the remaining pastries.
- ❖ Repeat until all the filling and phyllo strips are used up.
- ❖ Bake for 20 to 30 minutes until the triangles are crisp and golden.
- ❖ Serve hot, warm or cold.

34. BALSAMIC TOMATO VEGETABLE SALAD

Tomatoes, sweet onions, and cucumbers shine in a balsamic vinaigrette for a cool and refreshing salad. You may serve this over greens if you wish, but it's delicious just as is. Plan ahead for the vegetables to marinate a couple of hours before serving. Prep time is 2 hours and 15 minutes as a whole providing you with about 6 portions.

Ingredients:

1/4 cup balsamic vinegar
1/4 cup sweet red wine (such as Lambrusco)
1/8 cup water
1/4 cup olive oil
1 tablespoon Dijon mustard
1 clove garlic, peeled and forced through a press
1/8 teaspoon salt
Pinch of sugar, optional
Freshly ground black pepper to taste
3 small tomatoes cut into wedges
1 medium sweet onion (such as Vidalia), sliced into 1/4-inch thick rings
1 cucumber, sliced into 1/4-inch thick rounds
6 fresh basil leaves sliced into 1/8-inch ribbons (chiffonade)
Parmesan cheese for garnish, optional

✱ Preparation:

Make the Vinaigrette:

❖ Whisk together balsamic vinegar, red wine, water, olive oil, Dijon mustard, garlic, sugar (if using), salt, and pepper until combined.

Then:

- ❖ Place tomatoes, onion, cucumber, and basil in a zip-top bag.
- ❖ Cover with vinaigrette.
- ❖ Squeeze out the air from the bag and seal. Toss to coat.
- ❖ Chill in the refrigerator at least two hours.
- ❖ Sprinkle with grated Parmesan cheese just before serving if desired.

35. THREE CHEESE PENNE PASTA

Cheese, garlic, and mushrooms star in this low-fat pasta dish. Prep time is 15 minutes while cook time is 30 minutes for a total time of 45 minutes yielding you 8 servings.

Ingredients:

1 pound whole wheat penne
2 tablespoons olive oil
1 pound mushrooms, sliced
1 large onion, chopped
2 cloves garlic, finely chopped
1/4 cup all-purpose flour
4 cups low-fat (1%) milk
1/2 teaspoon salt
1/4 teaspoon ground nutmeg
4 teaspoons fresh lemon juice
1/4 teaspoon black pepper
1-1/2 cups shredded reduced-fat cheddar cheese (6 ounces)
1-1/4 cups shredded reduced-fat Swiss cheese (5 ounces)
1 cup shredded reduced-fat Monterey Jack cheese (4 ounces)

✳ How to prepare:

- ❖ Cook penne in a large pot of lightly salted boiling water until al dente, firm but tender.
- ❖ Drain well.
- ❖ Meanwhile, heat 1 tablespoon olive oil in a large skillet over medium-high heat.
- ❖ Add mushrooms, saute 8 minutes or until tender.
- ❖ Remove form skillet.
- ❖ Heat remaining oil in skillet.
- ❖ Add onion, saute 5 minutes.
- ❖ Add garlic; saute 2 minutes.
- ❖ Whisk together flour and milk in a small bowl.
- ❖ Add to skillet.
- ❖ Bring to boiling, stirring occasionally.

- ❖ Reduce heat to low; add salt and nutmeg and simmer 5 minutes.
- ❖ Heat oven to 400 degrees F.
- ❖ Lighly grease a 12 x 9 x 2-inch shallow baking dish.
- ❖ In same pot used to cook penne, toss penne with sauce, mushrooms, lemon juice and pepper.
- ❖ Combine all the cheddar, Swiss, and Monterey Jack cheeses in a bowl; set aside 1/4 cup.
- ❖ Add remaining cheese to penne mixture, stirring gently.
- ❖ Spoon into prepared baking dish.
- ❖ Sprinkle with reserved cheese.
- ❖ Bake, uncovered, in heated 400-degree F. oven, 20 to 30 minutes or until browned and bubbly.
- ❖ Make-ahead tip: Prepare through all steps except baking.
- ❖ Refrigerate, covered, up to 3 days or freeze up to 1 month.
- ❖ To serve, if frozen, thaw in refrigerator overnight.
- ❖ Bake as directed.

36. TROPICAL COUSCOUS

Citrus juices, mango, fresh ginger, and herbs give a tropical flair to couscous. This pasta dish is incredibly fast and easy to make. It is served at room temperature so it's a great choice for buffets and parties. Prep time is 10 minutes while cook time is only 5 minutes for a total time of just 15 minutes providing you with 8 portions.

Ingredients:

2-1/4 cups fresh orange juice
1 tsp ground cumin
1 box (10 ounces) couscous
2 Tbsp olive oil
2 Tbsp reduced-sodium soy sauce
2 Tbsp fresh lime juice
1/4 cup chopped fresh cilantro
2 Tbsp chopped fresh basil or 1 tsp dried
2 Tbsp chopped fresh chives
1 tsp grated fresh ginger
1 mango, peeled, pitted and chopped
1/4 cup pine nuts, toasted

✳ How to prepare:

- ❖ Bring orange juice and cumin to boiling in a medium-size saucepan.
- ❖ Add couscous and cover.
- ❖ Remove from heat and let stand 5 minutes.
- ❖ Remove to a large bowl; cool.
- ❖ Mix olive oil, soy sauce and lime juice in a small bowl.
- ❖ Stir into couscous.
- ❖ Stir in cilantro,basil, chives, ginger, mango, and orange.
- ❖ Sprinkle with pine nuts.

37.   VEGETABLE LASAGNA RECIPE

Loaded with mushrooms, broccoli, and olives, this lasagna is both low-fat and delicious. This lasagna may be made up to 2 days in advance. Prep time is 20 minutes and cook time clocks in at about 1 hour for a total time of 1 hour and 20 minutes yielding 6 servings.

Ingredients:

1 Tablespoon olive oil
1/2 large onion, chopped
3 cups sliced mushrooms
2 cloves roasted garlic, minced
3 cups broccoli florets, blanched
1/4 cup sliced black olives
1 cup low-fat ricotta cheese
1/2 cup silken tofu
2 Tablespoons packed soy protein powder
1/4 teaspoon oregano
1/4 teaspoon basil
1 (8-ounce) package whole wheat lasagna noodles
3 cups tomato sauce
12 ounces shredded soy mozzarella

✳ How to prepare:

- ❖ Preheat oven to 350 F.
- ❖ Heat olive oil in a nonstick skillet; add onion and cook until soft, about 5 minutes.
- ❖ Add mushrooms and garlic and cook until mushrooms are soft, about 3 minutes longer.
- ❖ Remove from heat and add broccoli and olives.
- ❖ Mix gently.
- ❖ Combine ricotta cheese, tofu, soy protein powder, oregano, and basil in a medium bowl until blended.
- ❖ Bring 4 quarts water and 1/2 teaspoon olive oil to a boil.

- ❖ Add lasagna noodles and boil 12 minutes or until tender.
- ❖ Drain and rinse under warm water.
- ❖ Moisten the bottom of a 9 x 9-inch pan with 2 tablespoons of the tomato sauce.
- ❖ Put down a single layer of noodles.
- ❖ Spread with one-third of the ricotta mix, one-third of the vegetables, 2/3 cup tomato sauce, and one-fourth of the mozzarella.
- ❖ Repeat twice.
- ❖ Cover with remaining noodles, tomato sauce, and mozzarella.
- ❖ Bake in a preheated oven for 45 minutes or until bubbling.

38. YUKON GOLD POTATO AND ARTICHOKE SALAD

Red onions, olives, basil, and lemon accent this unusual potato salad using gold potatoes and artichokes. Prep time is only 20 minutes while cook time is 30 minutes for a total time of 50 minutes providing you with 6 portions.

Ingredients:

Salad:

8 medium Yukon Gold potatoes (about 2 3/4 pounds)
1 lemon, halved
4 large artichokes
1-2/3 cups water
1/3 cup olive oil
1/3 cup dry white wine
6 whole black peppercorns
6 coriander seeds
2 fresh thyme sprigs or 1/2 teaspoon dried
1/2 red onion, very thinly sliced
3 green onions, thinly sliced diagonally
1 tomato, peeled, seeded, chopped
10 black brine-cured olives (such a Nicois or Kalamata), pitted, chopped
6 fresh basil leaves, thinly sliced

Dressing:

1/4 cup fresh lemon juice
2 Tablespoons Dijon mustard
3/4 cup olive oil

✳ How to prepare:

Make Salad:

- ❖ Cook gold potatoes in large pot of boiling salted water until just tender, about 22 minutes.
- ❖ Drain well. Cool.
- ❖ Cut into 1-inch pieces.
- ❖ Halfway fill large bowl with cold water.
- ❖ Squeeze in juice from half of lemon.
- ❖ Cut second lemon half in half.
- ❖ Cut off stem from 1 artichoke and rub exposed area with cut side of lemon piece.
- ❖ Starting from base of artichoke, bend each leaf back and snap off where leaf breaks naturally.
- ❖ Continue until light green leaves are exposed.
- ❖ Cut off top 2 inches of artichoke above heart.
- ❖ Using small sharp knife, cut off all dark green areas.
- ❖ Cut artichoke heart into quarters.
- ❖ Rub all cut surfaces with lemon piece.
- ❖ Cut out choke and pink inner leaves from each section and discard.
- ❖ Place artichoke heart sections in water with lemon juice.
- ❖ Repeat with remaining artichokes.
- ❖ Combine 1-2/3 cups water, olive oil, wine, peppercorns, coriander, and thyme in heavy large saucepan and bring to boil.
- ❖ Drain artichokes.
- ❖ Add to saucepan.
- ❖ Cook until tender, about 15 minutes.
- ❖ Drain. Cool.
- ❖ Cut into slices. (Potatoes and artichokes can be made 1 day ahead. Cover separately and refrigerate.)
- ❖ Mix potatoes, artichoke slices, Red onions, green onions, tomato, olives, and basil in large bowl.

Make Dressing:

- ❖ Mix lemon juice and mustard in medium bowl.
- ❖ Gradually whisk in olive oil.
- ❖ Mix into salad. S
- ❖ Season to taste with sea salt and pepper.

39.   APPLE ORANGE RAISIN SALAD

A simple salad recipe that takes 5 minutes to prepare and will yield you 4 to 6 servings.

Ingredients:

4 Gala apples, cut into chunks
2 navel oranges, cut into chunks
2 tablespoons raisins
1 tablespoon of olive oil

* How to prepare:

- ❖ In a bowl, combine the apples, oranges, raisins, and oil.
- ❖ Press some oranges with the back of a spoon to release juice.
- ❖ Cover and refrigerate for about 1 hour.
- ❖ Allow to sit at room temperature 10 minutes before tossing and serving.

40.   BRUSSEL SPROUTS IN TOMATO SAUCE

A quick recipe takes about 10 minutes prep time and 15 minutes cook time for a total of 25 minutes providing you with 5 servings.

Ingredients:

2 tablespoons of Olive oil

1 1/4 pounds Brussels sprouts, quartered

1 can (8 ounces) tomato purée

2 cloves garlic, minced

1/2 teaspoon salt

✳ How to prepare:

- ❖ In a large sauté pan, heat the oil.
- ❖ Add the Brussels sprouts.
- ❖ Cover and cook for about 3 minutes, turning occasionally, or until they start to brown.
- ❖ Add the tomato purée, garlic, and salt.
- ❖ Stir.
- ❖ Cover and reduce the heat to low.
- ❖ Cook for about 8 minutes, or until the Brussels sprouts are tender.

41. FENNEL SALAD

A simple salad that will take you about 5-10 minutes to prepare and will yield you about 4 servings.

Ingredients:

1 medium bulb fennel
2 tablespoons (1/2 ounce) grated Parmesan cheese
1 tablespoon olive oil
2 teaspoons Red Wine Vinegar or white wine vinegar
1/4 teaspoon ground black pepper

✱ How to prepare:

- ❖ Cut the top stalks from the fennel bulb.
- ❖ Reserve some of the dill-like leaves; discard the stalks.
- ❖ Cut the fennel into lengthwise quarters.
- ❖ Cut out and discard the core sections.
- ❖ Cut the quarters into thin slices.
- ❖ Chop the leaves.
- ❖ Place in a bowl with the cheese, oil, vinegar, and pepper.
- ❖ Toss to mix. Enjoy!

42. ORANGE-GLAZED ROASTED SALMON AND FENNEL

This delicious recipe takes about 20 minutes of prep time and 40 minutes of cooking time for a total of 1 hour of your time, yielding you 4 to 6 servings.

Ingredients:

2 to 3 navel oranges
2 tablespoons Olive Oil, plus some for the baking pan
1 1/2 teaspoons salt
2 large bulbs fennel
1 large salmon fillet (2 to 2 1/2 pounds)

✻ How to prepare:

- ❖ Preheat the oven to 400°F.
- ❖ Coat a 16 x 10-inch baking pan with oil.
- ❖ Grate 1 tablespoon orange zest.
- ❖ Squeeze oranges to get 1/2 cup juice.
- ❖ In a small bowl whisk the zest, juice, oil, and salt.
- ❖ Trim the fennel.
- ❖ Mince about 2 tablespoons of the feathery leaves; set aside. (The remaining leaves may be reserved for salads or other recipes.)
- ❖ Cut bulbs lengthwise into quarters.
- ❖ Cut out and discard the cores.
- ❖ Cut the fennel into thick slices.
- ❖ Place the fennel in the baking pan.
- ❖ Drizzle with half of the juice mixture.
- ❖ Toss to coat.
- ❖ Place in the oven for about 20 minutes, stirring occasionally, or until lightly browned.
- ❖ Remove the pan from the oven.
- ❖ Clear a space in the center and lay the salmon diagonally in the pan, skin side down.
- ❖ Drizzle with the remaining juice mixture.
- ❖ Spread to coat the fish.

❖ Place in the oven and roast for about 15 minutes, or until the salmon is opaque in the center.

43.   SKILLET PIZZA

This simple pizza dish takes about 15 minutes prep time and about 15-20 minutes cooking time depending how golden you like your crust for a total of 30-35 minutes providing you with about 2 9-10 inch pizzas.

Ingredients:

1 pound store-bought whole wheat pizza dough, at room temperature

1 medium ripe tomato, thinly sliced

1/4 pound fresh mozzarella cheese, cut into bits

2 tablespoons Olive Oil, plus some for pan

1/2 cup shredded fresh basil leaves

some sea salt

✳ How to prepare:

❖ Heat a well-oiled cast-iron 10-or 12-inch frying pan for 5 minutes over medium heat. If you don't have a cast-iron pan, use a nonstick pan.

❖ Divide the dough in half and roll the dough into a circle one inch smaller than the diameter of the pan you are using.

❖ Place the dough in the hot pan and allow it to cook until it begins to rise and the bottom starts to brown.

❖ Carefully flip the dough over with a metal spatula.

❖ Lay half the tomato slices over the dough and scatter half the cheese over the tomatoes.

❖ Lower the heat to medium-low and continue to cook the pizza until the cheese has melted.

❖ Use a metal spatula to transfer the pizza to cutting board.

❖ Sprinkle the pizza with salt and drizzle with olive oil.

❖ Cut into wedges and sprinkle half the basil over the wedges. à

❖ Repeat for second pizza.

44. TABBOULEH SALAD

A popular salad that I enjoy with whole wheat pita bread, takes about 20 minutes to prepare including cooking time yielding about 4 portions.

Ingredients:

1 cup (250 mL) medium or coarse bulgur
1 can (19oz) drained and rinsed chickpeas
2 tomatoes, seeded and chopped
1 cup (250 mL) diced English cucumbers
1 cup (250 mL) minced fresh Italian parsley
1/2 cup (125 mL) chopped green onions
1/4 cup (60 mL) chopped fresh mint

Dressing:

1/4 cup (60 mL) lemon juice
2 tbsp (30 mL) olive oil
2 cloves of garlic, minced
1 tsp (5 mL)sea salt
1/2 tsp (2 mL) pepper

✳ How to prepare:

- ❖ In saucepan, bring 1-3/4 cups (425 mL) water to boil; stir in bulgur.
- ❖ Reduce heat to low; cover and cook for 10 minutes or until no liquid remains.
- ❖ Transfer to large bowl, fluffing with fork.
- ❖ Let cool to room temperature.
- ❖ Add chickpeas, tomatoes, cucumber, parsley, onions and mint.

Dressing:

In small bowl, whisk together lemon juice, oil, garlic, salt and pepper; pour over bulgur mixture and toss to combine.

45.   BARLEY SALAD WITH TOMATOES AND CORN

Barley is a source of B-complex vitamins and a good source of soluble fibre, this recipe is definitely gout friendly, prep time and cook time is about 1 hour and will yield you about 6 portions.

Ingredients:

1 cup (250 mL) pearl barley
1 cup (250 mL) tightly packed fresh basil leaves
1/3 cup (75 mL) grated Parmesan cheese
1/4 cup (60 mL) olive oil
1/2 tsp (2 mL) sea salt
1/2 tsp (2 mL) pepper
2 cloves garlic, minced
4 cups (1 L) cherry tomatoes, halved or about 5 medium-size tomatoes.
2 cups (500 mL) corn kernels, cooked (about 3 cobs)

✳ How to prepare:

❖ Bring large pot of water to boil; add barley.
❖ Reduce heat, cover and simmer, stirring occasionally, for about 50 minutes or until tender.
❖ Drain; chill under cold running water and drain again.
❖ Meanwhile, in food processor or blender, put basil, Parmesan, oil, salt and pepper; stir in garlic.
❖ Toss with barley.
❖ Add tomatoes and corn; toss again. *(Make ahead: Cover and refrigerate for up to 2 days.)*

46. BEET, ORANGE AND WATERCRESS SALAD

Sweet roasted beets get a fresh orange lift in this colourful salad with a tangy vinaigrette. Substitute a mixture of arugula, radicchio and fresh spinach for the watercress if you like. Prep time including cook time for this salad is about 1 hour and 30 minutes due to the cooking of the beets, once that is out of the way the rest takes a mere few minutes and will yield you 8 portions.

Ingredients:

6 unpeeled, trimmed beets, (1-1/2 lb/750 g)
2 oranges
2 bunches watercress
1/4 cup (60 mL) sliced almonds, toasted

Dressing:

1 tsp (5 mL) finely grated orange rind
2 tbsp (30 mL) orange juice
2 tbsp (30 mL) olive oil
1 tbsp (15 mL) white wine vinegar
1/2 tsp (2 mL) Dijon mustard
1/2 tsp (2 mL) granulated sugar
1 pinch each sea salt, and pepper

✳ How to prepare:

- ❖ Wrap beets in foil and roast in 400°F (200°C) oven for 1 to 1-1/2 hours or until tender. (Alternatively, cook beets in boiling water for about 40 minutes or until tender.)
- ❖ Let cool slightly; rub off skins and cut into thick slices.
- ❖ In small bowl, whisk together orange rind, orange juice, olive oil, vinegar, mustard, sugar, sea salt and pepper.

- ❖ (Make-ahead: Transfer beets to separate bowl; cover beets and dressing with plastic wrap. Refrigerate for up to 1 day.)
- ❖ With sharp knife, cut peel and pith off oranges; cut in half lengthwise, then slice crosswise, removing outer membrane.
- ❖ Remove tough stems from watercress.
- ❖ In shallow serving bowl, toss watercress with half of the dressing.
- ❖ Toss beets with remaining dressing and arrange in centre of watercress.
- ❖ Arrange oranges over watercress.
- ❖ Sprinkle almonds over top.

47. GRILLED VEGETABLE SALAD WITH TARRAGON DRESSING

This tasty grilled vegetable salad takes about 10 minutes of prep time and 10 minutes of cook time for the vegetables yielding you about 6 servings.

Ingredients:

1 yellow zucchini
1 green zucchini
1 sweet green pepper, cored
1 sweet red pepper, cored
1 large carrot, peeled
1 large eggplant
1/2 cup (125 mL) olive oil
2 cloves garlic, minced
1 jalapeño pepper, seeded and minced
1/4 tsp (1 mL) each sea salt, and pepper
1/4 cup (60 mL) sunflower seeds

Dressing:

1 tbsp (15 mL) chopped fresh tarragon
1 tbsp (15 mL) lemon juice
1 tbsp (15 mL) balsamic vinegar
1 tsp (5 mL) liquid honey
1 shallot, finely chopped
1 clove garlic, minced
1 pinch each sea salt and pepper
1/3 cup (75 mL) olive oil

✳ How to prepare:

- ❖ Cut both zucchini, both peppers, carrot and eggplant lengthwise into 1/2-inch (1 cm) thick slices.
- ❖ In large bowl, whisk together olive oil, garlic, jalapeno salt and pepper; add vegetables and toss to coat.
- ❖ Place vegetables, in batches, on greased grill over medium heat; close lid and cook, turning occasionally, for 10 minutes or just until tender-crisp.
- ❖ Let cool on cutting board; cut into 2- x 1/2-inch (5 x 1 cm) sticks.
- ❖ For the dressing, in large bowl, combine tarragon, lemon juice, vinegar, honey, shallot, garlic, salt and pepper; gradually whisk in oil.
- ❖ Add vegetables; stir to coat.
- ❖ Serve sprinkled with sunflower seeds.

48. GRAPEFRUIT, AVOCADO AND WATERCRESS SALAD

Tangy citrus dressing enlivens peppery watercress in this brunch salad, yes good for breakfast or a light lunch to get your day going. The prep and cook time is about 15-20 minutes here yielding you about 4 to 6 servings.

Ingredients:

3 ruby red grapefruits
1/4 cup (60 mL) olive oil
1/4 tsp (1 mL) sea salt
1/4 tsp (1 mL) pepper
1 avocado, peeled and sliced
1 bunch large watercress, coarse stems removed
2 cups (500 mL) torn radicchio lettuce
2 tbsp (30 mL) thinly sliced green onions

✳ How to prepare:

- ❖ With vegetable peeler, peel rind from 1 of the grapefruit.
- ❖ With knife, cut enough rind into long paper-thin strips (julienne) to make 1/4 cup (50 mL); set aside.
- ❖ Peel remaining grapefruit.
- ❖ Cut away white pith from all grapefruit.
- ❖ Working over sieve set over measuring cup or bowl, slice grapefruit between membranes and pulp to release sections; set aside.
- ❖ Squeeze membranes to make 1/2 cup (125 mL) juice.
- ❖ In small saucepan, cover reserved rind with water and bring to boil.
- ❖ Reduce heat and simmer until tender, about 1 minute; drain and add to grapefruit juice.
- ❖ Add olive oil, sea salt and pepper.
- ❖ If you wish (Make-ahead: Refrigerate dressing and grapefruit in separate airtight containers for up to 2 days.)
- ❖ Peel, pit and slice avocado.

- ❖ In bowl, toss watercress with radicchio.
- ❖ Top with grapefruit and avocado; drizzle with dressing.
- ❖ Sprinkle with onions.

49. MINTY WARM RICE AND VEGETABLE SALAD

This salad recipe is very easy to prepare taking you only 5-10 minutes prep time and 20 minutes cook time for a total of 30-35 minutes of your time yielding you 4 servings. You can also replace the rice for couscous instead.

Ingredients:

1-1/2 cups (375 mL) vegetable stock
3/4 cup (175 mL) long-grain rice
1 zucchini, grated
1 cup (250 mL) snow_peas, cut_in half
1 can (19 oz/540 mL) chickpeas, drained and rinsed
1 sweet red pepper, chopped
1/4 cup (50 mL) chopped fresh mint
2 tbsp (25 mL) wine_vinegar
1 tbsp (15 mL) olive_oil
1 clove garlic, minced
1/4 tsp (1 mL) each salt and pepper

✱ How to prepare:

- ❖ In saucepan, bring stock to boil.
- ❖ Add rice; cover and cook over low heat for 15 minutes.
- ❖ Add zucchini and snow peas; cook, covered, for 5 minutes or until rice is tender.
- ❖ Fluff with fork.
- ❖ Add chickpeas, red pepper, mint, vinegar, olive oil, garlic, sea salt and pepper; toss gently.

50.   CARROT AND LOTS OF GARLIC SOUP

This soup is so tasty that you may want to try it not only as a quick weeknight vegetarian supper (with crusty whole wheat bread and a salad) but also as a first course when entertaining. Prep time for this soup is about 20 minutes and cooking time about 35-40 minutes for a total time of about 1 hour providing you with 4 to 6 servings.

Ingredients:

2 heads garlic
1 tbsp (15 mL) extra virgin olive oil
1 onion, chopped
1/2 tsp (2 mL) sea salt
1/2 tsp (2 mL) pepper
5 cups (1.25 L) vegetable stock
3 cups (750 mL) chopped carrots
1 potato, peeled and chopped
1 cup (250 mL) shredded fresh basil
1/4 cup (60 mL) light sour cream or plain yogurt, optional
1/4 cup (60 mL) minced fresh chives

✳ How to prepare:

❖ Separate and peel garlic cloves.
❖ In large saucepan, heat oil over medium heat; fry garlic, onion, salt and pepper, stirring, until onion is softened, about 5 minutes.
❖ Add stock, carrots, potato and 1 cup (250 mL) water; bring to boil.
❖ Cover, reduce heat and simmer until vegetables are tender, about 20 minutes.
❖ Using immersion blender or in batches in blender, purée soup until smooth.
❖ Add water to thin, if desired.
❖ Stir in basil. Ladle into bowls; top with sour cream (if using) and chives.

51. LENTIL VEGETABLE SOUP

This traditional hearty soup features lentils, chickpeas, pasta and vegetables with aromatic yet mild spices. In Morocco its name is harira, and it serves to break the Ramadan fast in Muslim homes. Prep time for this savoury soup is about 15 minutes and cook time is about 6 hours and a half for a total time of about 7 hours but does yield you 10 to 12 portions but the taste is well worth the time not to mention all the gout friendly ingredients.

Ingredients:

1 tbsp (15 mL) olive oil
4 celery stalks, with leaves, chopped
2 onions, chopped
2 tsp (10 mL) cinnamon
2 tsp (10 mL) ground cumin
2 tsp (10 mL) ground ginger
2 tsp (10 mL) pepper
2 tsp (10 mL) turmeric
2 cans (each 10 oz/284 mL) vegetable stock
1 can (28 oz/796 mL) diced tomatoes
2 cups (500 mL) diced peeled seeded squash
3/4 cup (175 mL) green lentils or brown lentils
1 can (19 oz/540 mL) chickpeas, drained and rinsed
1 cup (250 mL) cooked small pasta or rice
1 zucchini, diced
1/4 cup (60 mL) fresh parsley, chopped
1/4 cup (60 mL) fresh coriander, chopped
1/4 cup (60 mL) lemon juice

✱ How to prepare:

- ❖ In large skillet, heat oil over medium heat; fry celery, onions, cinnamon, cumin, ginger, pepper and turmeric until onions are softened, about 5 minutes.
- ❖ Scrape into slow-cooker.
- ❖ Add vegetable stock, tomatoes, squash, lentils and 4 cups (1 L) water.
- ❖ Cover and cook on low until squash is tender, about 6 hours.
- ❖ Stir in chickpeas, pasta and zucchini.
- ❖ Increase heat to high; cover and cook until pasta is hot and zucchini is softened, about 25 minutes.
- ❖ Stir in parsley, coriander and lemon juice.

52.   LIMA BEAN TOMATO SOUP

This simple soup recipe takes about 10 minutes of prep time and 20 minutes of cook time for a total of 30 minutes of your time and will provide you with 4 portions.

Ingredients:

1 tbsp (15 mL) extra-virgin olive oil
1 onion, finely chopped
4 garlic cloves, minced
1/4 tsp (1 mL) hot pepper flakes
28 oz (794 g) diced tomatoes
3-1/2 cups (875 mL) vegetable stock
1 lb (454 g) frozen lima beans
2 tbsp (30 mL) chopped fresh parsley
1/4 tsp (1 mL) sea salt
1/4 cup (60 mL) grated romano cheese or Parmesan

✳ How to prepare:

- ❖ In large saucepan, heat oil over medium heat; cook onion, garlic and hot pepper flakes until softened, 5 minutes.
- ❖ Add tomatoes, stock and lima beans; bring to boil.
- ❖ Cover and reduce heat to medium-low; cook for 10 minutes.
- ❖ Add parsley and salt.
- ❖ Serve sprinkled with cheese.

53. PEAR AND CELERY SOUP

Silky-smooth, with the subtle flavours of pear and celery, every spoonful is a delight in this soup that's elegant enough for entertaining. Prep time is about 15 minutes and cooking time is about 40 minutes for a total time of 55 minutes yielding you about 8 servings.

Ingredients:

3 tbsp (45 mL) butter
5 cups (1.25 L) finely chopped celery
4 onions, sliced
1/4 cup (60 mL) minced fresh chives
1/2 tsp (2 mL) dried thyme
1/2 tsp (2 mL) sea salt
1/4 tsp (1 mL) pepper
6 cups (1.5 L) vegetable stock
3 pears, peeled, cored and sliced
1/2 cup (125 mL) 10% cream

✱ How to prepare:

- ❖ In saucepan, melt butter over medium heat.
- ❖ Cook celery, onions, chives, thyme, salt and pepper, covered and stirring occasionally, for about 10 minutes or until softened and translucent.
- ❖ Pour in stock; bring to boil.
- ❖ Reduce heat and simmer for 10 minutes or until celery is very tender.
- ❖ Add pears; cook for 5 minutes or until pears are tender.
- ❖ In batches, purée in blender.
- ❖ Return to saucepan; pour in cream and heat through without boiling.

54.   BROCCOLI AND CHEESE SOUFFLE

Cheese is always an excellent complement to broccoli. Wheel-shaped Gouda has a light yellow body and usually a golden orange wax rind. This recipe provides you with 4 portions and takes about 15 minutes of prep time and about 1 hour and 15 minutes of cooking time. This recipe can be used also as a side dish.

Ingredients:

2 cups (500 mL) chopped broccoli florets
1/4 cup (60 mL) butter
1/4 cup (60 mL) whole wheat flour
1/2 tsp (2 mL) dried thyme
1/4 tsp (1 mL) pepper
1 cup (250 mL) milk
1-1/2 cups (375 mL) shredded Gouda cheese, (6 oz/175 g)
4 eggs, separated

✳ How to prepare:

- ❖ In pot of boiling salted water, cook broccoli for 2 minutes or until tender-crisp.
- ❖ Drain and chill under cold running water.
- ❖ In saucepan, melt butter over medium heat; cook flour, thyme and pepper, stirring, for 1 minute.
- ❖ Gradually pour in milk; cook, stirring, for about 5 minutes or until smooth and very thick.
- ❖ Remove from heat; stir in cheese until almost melted.
- ❖ Whisk 1/2 cup (125 mL) of the cheese mixture into egg yolks.
- ❖ Whisk back into saucepan.
- ❖ Fold in broccoli.
- ❖ Let cool completely. (Souffle be prepared to this point, covered and refrigerated for up to 12 hours. Cover and refrigerate egg whites; let come to room temperature.)
- ❖ Beat egg whites until stiff peaks form; fold one-quarter of the whites into broccoli mixture; fold in remaining whites.

- ❖ Spoon into 6- x 3-inch or 7- x 3-inch (1 L or 1.5 L) souffle-ish. B

❖ Bake in 350°F (180°C) oven for about 1 hour or until golden brown and tester inserted in centre comes out clean.

55.   CHEESY PITA POCKETS

This lunch, a combination of carbohydrates (from the whole grain pita) and protein (from the cheese) will help you store energy to use later in the day, thereby dispelling that late-afternoon urge to doze. Prep time for this simple recipe is about 10 minutes with no cooking required and will provide you with 2 portions.

Ingredients:

1/3 cup (75 mL) light cream cheese, softened
1/4 cup (60 mL) shredded old Cheddar cheese
1 carrot, shredded
1/4 tsp (1 mL) pepper
1 whole wheat pita bread
1/4 large cucumber, sliced
1/2 cup (125 mL) alfalfa sprouts or radish sprouts or onion sprouts

✳ How to prepare:

* ❖ In small bowl, mash together cream and Cheddar cheeses, shredded carrot and pepper until blended.
* ❖ Cut top quarter of each pita and tuck inside bottom of pita.
* ❖ Spread half of the cheese mixture inside each; fill with cucumber and sprouts.

56. BLACK BEAN QUESADILLAS

Beans are packed with both soluble and insoluble fibre, which can help to keep your digestive system regular, regulate blood sugar, lower cholesterol and protect against some cancers. Prep time for this recipe is about 10 minutes and cook time is about 30 minutes for a total of 40 minutes providing you with 4 servings.

Ingredients:

2 tsp (10 mL) olive oil
1 chopped onion
1 diced sweet green pepper
1 tbsp (15 mL) chili powder
1/2 tsp (2 mL) ground cumin
1/4 tsp (1 mL) sea salt
1/4 tsp (1 mL) pepper
1 can (19oz) black beans, drained and rinsed
1 cup (250 mL) salsa
1/2 cup (125 mL) corn kernels
4 large flour tortillas
2 cups (500 mL) shredded Cheddar cheese
1/2 cup (125 mL) sour cream, light
1/4 cup (60 mL) diced fresh jalapeño peppers or pickled jalapeño peppers, optional

✱ How to prepare:

* ❖ In large nonstick skillet, heat oil over medium heat; cook onion, green pepper, chili powder, cumin, salt and pepper until softened, about 8 minutes.
* ❖ Add black beans, salsa and corn; cook, stirring often, until heated through, about 5 minutes.
* ❖ Evenly spoon bean mixture over half of each tortilla; sprinkle with cheese.
* ❖ Fold uncovered half over top and press lightly.
* ❖ Place on large rimmed baking sheet; bake in 425°F (220°C) oven, turning once, until golden, 10 to 15 minutes.
* ❖ Serve with sour cream, and jalapeno peppers (if using).

57. BUCATINI WITH ROASTED GARLIC AND CHERRY TOMATOES

Roasting tomatoes brings out their rich flavour, and using cherry tomatoes speeds up the process. The harshness of the garlic mellows during roasting. For the Parmesan, a piece of Parmigiano-Reggiano has the best flavour and shaves nicely over the pasta. You can substitute other sharp hard cheeses, such as Grana Padano, Romano or Asiago. Prep time is about 20 minutes while cook time is about 45 minutes for a total of 1 hour and 5 minutes of your time yielding you 5 servings.

Ingredients:

4 cups (1 L) cherry tomatoes, halved

12 cloves garlic, halved

1/4 cup (50 mL) extra-virgin olive oil

1 tsp (5 mL) dried basil

1/2 tsp (2 mL) sea salt

1/4 tsp (1 mL) hot pepper flakes

1/4 tsp (1 mL) pepper

1 lb (500 g) bucatini pasta

1/4 cup (60 mL) chopped fresh parsley

1/2 cup (125 mL) shaved Parmesan cheese

✴ How to prepare:

- ❖ In 13- x 9-inch (3.5 L) metal cake pan, toss together tomatoes, garlic, oil, basil, salt, hot pepper flakes and pepper; roast in 400°F (200°C) oven until tomatoes are shrivelled and garlic is tender, about 30 minutes.
- ❖ Meanwhile, in large pot of boiling salted water, cook pasta until tender but firm, 8 to 10 minutes.
- ❖ Drain and return to pot.
- ❖ Add tomato mixture and parsley, tossing to coat.
- ❖ Serve sprinkled with Parmesan.

58. EGGPLANT AND POTATO RAGOUT WITH FETA TOPPING

This savoury dish will take you about 20 minutes of prep time and 1 hour and 30 minutes of cooking time but well worth it and will yield you 8 portions.

Ingredients:

1-1/2 lb (680 g) eggplant, cut into 3/4-inch (2 cm) cubes
2 tsp (10 mL) sea salt
1/3 cup (75 mL) extra-virgin olive oil
4 (2 lb/1 kg) Yukon Gold potatoes, unpeeled and cut into 3/4-inch (2 cm) cubes
12 oz (340 g) sliced mushrooms, (about 4 cups/ 1L)
1 large onion, chopped
6 cloves garlic, minced
1 tbsp (15 mL) dried oregano
1/2 tsp (2 mL) dried basil
1/2 tsp (2 mL) pepper
1 sweet red pepper, chopped
1 sweet green pepper, chopped
2 cans (each 19 oz/540 mL) stewed tomatoes
1 cup (250 mL) vegetable stock
1/4 cup (60 mL) tomato paste

Feta Topping:

2-1/2 cups (625 mL) fresh bread crumbs
1-3/4 cups (425 mL) crumbled feta cheese
1/4 cup (60 mL) chopped oil-cured black olives
1/4 cup (60 mL) chopped Italian parsley
1 tsp (5 mL) dried oregano

✳ How to prepare:

- ❖ In colander, sprinkle eggplant with 1 tsp (5 mL) of the salt ; set aside.
- ❖ Meanwhile, in large deep Dutch oven, heat 3 tbsp (50 mL) of the oil over medium-high heat; brown potatoes.
- ❖ Remove potatoes to plate.
- ❖ Rinse eggplant; pat dry.
- ❖ Add half of the remaining oil to pan; brown eggplant, in 2 batches and adding remaining oil as necessary.
- ❖ Add to potatoes.
- ❖ In same skillet over medium-high heat, saute mushrooms, onion, garlic, oregano, basil, pepper and remaining salt until no liquid remains, about 8 minutes.
- ❖ Add red and green peppers; saute until beginning to brown, about 5 minutes.
- ❖ Add eggplant mixture, tomatoes, stock and tomato paste; bring to boil.
- ❖ Reduce heat and simmer until potatoes are tender, about 40 minutes.
- ❖ Meanwhile, in bowl, combine bread crumbs, feta cheese, olives, parsley and oregano.
- ❖ Spread over eggplant mixture; bake in 375°F (190°C) oven until bubbly and golden, about 25 minutes.

59.   WILD RICE AND BROCCOLI CASSEROLE

Great vegetarian dish which serves up 8 portions takes about 25 minutes of prep time and 2 hours of cooking time for a total of 2 hours and 25 minutes, it makes a great lunch recipe for work or even for a potluck event.

Ingredients:

1/4 cup (60 mL) wild rice, rinsed
1 cup (250 mL) parboiled white rice
5 cups (1.25 L) broccoli florets
1 tbsp (15 mL) butter
1 onion, chopped
1 clove garlic, minced
4 cups (1 L) sliced mushrooms, (about 10 oz/300 g)
1-1/2 tsp (7 mL) dried thyme
3/4 tsp (4 mL) pepper
1/2 tsp (2 mL) sea salt
1/3 cup (75 mL) whole wheat flour
2-1/4 cups (550 mL) vegetable stock
1/2 cup (125 mL) 18% cream
1-1/2 cups (375 mL) shredded old Cheddar cheese
1/2 cup (125 mL) fresh bread crumbs

✳ How to prepare:

- ❖ In saucepan, bring 3-1/2 cups (875 mL) water to boil; add wild rice and return to boil.
- ❖ Reduce heat, cover and simmer for 40 minutes.
- ❖ Stir in white rice; simmer, covered, for 20 minutes or until tender.
- ❖ Fluff with fork.
- ❖ Stir in broccoli; cook, covered, for about 5 minutes or until broccoli is tender-crisp.
- ❖ Meanwhile, in separate saucepan, melt butter over medium-high heat; cook onion, garlic, mushrooms, thyme, pepper and salt, stirring, for about 7 minutes or until softened and starting to brown.

- ❖ Sprinkle with flour; cook, stirring, for 1 minute.
- ❖ Gradually whisk in vegetable stock and cream; bring to boil, stirring.
- ❖ Reduce heat and simmer, stirring, for 5 minutes or until thickened.
- ❖ Add to rice mixture along with 1/2 cup (125 mL) of the cheese.
- ❖ Transfer to 13- x 9-inch (3 L) baking dish. *(Casserole can be prepared to this point, covered with plastic wrap and refrigerated for up to 24 hours.)*
- ❖ Mix remaining cheese with bread crumbs; sprinkle over casserole.
- ❖ Cover with foil; bake in 350°F (180°C) oven for 30 minutes or until bubbly.
- ❖ Uncover and broil for 2 to 3 minutes or until golden.

60.   VEGETARIAN CABBAGE ROLLS

One of my favorite dishes, you'll enjoy this tasty recipe which takes about 20 minutes of prep time and about 3 hours of cooking time, mostly the 2 hours of baking at the end of the cooking for a grand total of 3 hours and 20 minutes of your time which yields you 6 servings.

Ingredients:

1 cabbage, (5 lb/22 kg)
1-1/2 tsp (7 mL) olive oil
1 onion, chopped
1 clove garlic, minced
1 tsp (5 mL) dried marjoram or dried oregano
1/2 tsp (2 mL) dried thyme
1/4 tsp (1 mL) caraway seeds, crushed (optional)
1 cup (250 mL) long-grain brown rice
2 cups (500 mL) vegetable stock
1 carrot, grated
1 zucchini, grated
1/4 tsp (1 mL) sea salt
1/4 tsp (1 mL) pepper
1 egg, beaten
1 can (28 oz/796 mL) sauerkraut, drained
1/4 cup (60 mL) tomato paste
2-1/2 cups (625 mL) tomato juice

✱ How to prepare:

❖ Remove core from cabbage.
❖ In large pot of boiling salted water, cover and cook cabbage for 8 to 10 minutes or until leaves are softened and easy to remove.
❖ Chill in cold water.
❖ Carefully remove 12 leaves, returning cabbage to pan for 2 to 3 minutes if leaves become difficult to remove.

❖ Drain on towels.
❖ Pare off coarse veins; set leaves aside.
❖ In saucepan, heat oil over medium heat; cook onion, garlic, marjoram, thyme, and caraway seeds (if using) for 5 minutes or until softened.
❖ Stir in rice.
❖ Add stock and bring to boil; reduce heat,, cover and simmer for 20 minutes or until rice is tender.
❖ Stir in carrot, zucchini, salt and pepper.
❖ Let cool to room temperature.
❖ Stir in egg.
❖ Spoon about 1/3 cup (75 mL) onto each leaf just above stem.
❖ Fold bottom and sides over filling; roll up.
❖ Line 13- x 9-inch (3 L) baking dish with half of the sauerkraut.
❖ Arrange cabbage rolls on top; cover with remaining sauerkraut.
❖ Whisk tomato paste into tomato juice; pour over rolls.
❖ Cover with foil; bake in 350°F (180°C) oven for 2 hours or until tender.
❖ Enjoy!

61. TEX MEX VEGETARIAN SHEPHERD'S PIE

Everybody loves shepherd's pie but here you can enjoy it without any red meat that is bad for your gout. Prep time for this recipe is about 20 minutes and cook time is about 1 hour and 20 minutes for a total of 1 hour and 40 minutes.

Ingredients:

2 lb (about 6) Yukon Gold potatoes, peeled
1/4 cup (60 mL) milk
1/4 cup (60 mL) butter
3/4 tsp (4 mL) sea salt
3/4 tsp (4 mL) pepper
1 tbsp (15 mL) olive oil
2 carrots, diced
1 onion, chopped
1 sweet green pepper, chopped
1 tbsp (15 mL) chili powder
1/2 tsp (2 mL) ground cumin
1 pinch cayenne pepper
3/4 cup (175 mL) bulgur
2 tbsp (30 mL) whole wheat flour
1-1/2 cups (375 mL) vegetable stock
1 cup (250 mL) corn kernels
2 tbsp (30 mL) chopped fresh parsley or pumpkin seeds

✱ How to prepare:

❖ Cut potatoes into 2-inch (5 cm) chunks.
❖ In saucepan of boiling water, cook potatoes for about 20 minutes or until tender but not mushy; drain and mash.
❖ Blend in milk, butter and 1/2 teaspoon (2 mL) each of the salt and pepper.
❖ Meanwhile, in large skillet, heat oil over medium heat.

- Add carrots, onion, green pepper, chili powder, cumin and cayenne; cook, stirring occasionally, for 5 minutes or until onion is softened.
- Add bulgur and flour; cook, stirring, for 1 minute.
- Gradually pour in stock.
- Reduce heat to low; cover and cook for 10 minutes or until liquid is absorbed.
- Add corn and remaining salt and pepper.
- Spread in 8-inch (2 L) square glass baking dish; spread mashed potatoes over top.
- Sprinkle with parsley.
- Bake in 350°F (180°C) oven for about 30 minutes or until filling is bubbling.
- Broil for 2 minutes or until light golden.

62. SQUASH AND KALE PHYLLO PIE

This recipe can be eaten as an entree, hearty side dish even as a light lunch. Prep time will take you 20 minutes roughly and about 1 hour and 15 minutes of cooking time for a total of 1 hour and 35 minutes yielding you 8 servings.

Ingredients:

1/4 cup (60 mL) pine nuts or slivered almonds
1/2 bunch kale
2 tbsp (30 mL) extra-virgin olive oil
4 green onions, chopped
3 cloves garlic, minced
3/4 tsp (4 mL) each sea salt and pepper
1 onion, chopped
4 cups (1 L) cubed peeled butternut squash
1/2 tsp (2 mL) crumbled dried sage
1/2 cup (125 mL) grated Parmesan cheese
2 tbsp (30 mL) dry bread crumbs
2 tbsp (30 mL) chopped fresh parsley
8 sheets phyllo pastry
1/2 cup (125 mL) butter, melted

✳ How to prepare:

- ❖ In small skillet, toast pine nuts over medium-low heat until light brown, about 8 minutes.
- ❖ On cutting board, trim off stems and centre ribs of kale; discard.
- ❖ Coarsely chop leaves to make 12 cups (3 L). Set aside.
- ❖ In large skillet, heat half of the oil over medium heat; fry green onions and half each of the garlic, salt and pepper until softened, about 5 minutes.
- ❖ Add half of the chopped kale and 1/2 cup (125 mL) water; cook, stirring, until slightly wilted, about 1 minute.
- ❖ Add remaining kale; cook, stirring frequently, until tender and liquid is evaporated, about 10 minutes.

- ❖ Stir in toasted pine nuts. Set aside.
- ❖ In large skillet, heat remaining oil over medium heat; fry onion with remaining garlic, salt and pepper, stirring occasionally, until softened, about 5 minutes.
- ❖ Add squash and sage; fry until squash is tender, about 8 minutes.
- ❖ Stir in Parmesan cheese, bread crumbs and parsley. Let cool.
- ❖ Lightly butter 9-inch (2.5 L) springform pan.
- ❖ Lightly brush 1 sheet of phyllo with butter, keeping remaining phyllo covered with damp towel to prevent drying out.
- ❖ Line up short end of phyllo sheet with centre of pan and lay in pan, fitting over bottom and up sides and leaving overhang.
- ❖ Lay second sheet of buttered phyllo next to but generously overlapping first sheet.
- ❖ Repeat with remaining 6 sheets of phyllo, overlapping each to cover bottom of pan.
- ❖ Spoon in half of the kale mixture; top with squash mixture and remaining kale.
- ❖ Fold phyllo overhang over filling; brush top with butter and tuck in edge.
- ❖ Bake in centre of 400°F (200°C) oven until crispy and golden brown, about 25 minutes.
- ❖ Let pie cool on rack for 10 minutes.

63. RISOTTO PRIMAVERA

Remember that Risotto is most fluid and creamy immediately after it has finished cooking, so if you're not serving it right away, stir in 1/2 cup (125 mL) additional stock or water before reheating. Prep time for this dish is about 10 minutes and cook time clocks in at about 40 minutes for a total of 50 minutes yielding you about 2-3 portions. I love risotto!

Ingredients:

12 oz (340 g) asparagus

1 cup (250 mL) low-sodium chicken stock or vegetable stock

1/4 tsp (1 mL) crumbled saffron, (optional)

2 tbsp (30 mL) butter

1/2 onion, diced

1 carrot, diced

1 small zucchini, diced

1/4 tsp (1 mL) each sea salt and pepper

3/4 cup (175 mL) arborio rice

1/2 cup (125 mL) white wine

1/2 cup (125 mL) fresh peas or frozen peas

1/4 cup (60 mL) grated Parmesan cheese

2 tbsp (30 mL) choppped fresh parsley

✳ How to prepare:

* ❖ Snap off woody ends of asparagus; cut into 1-inch (2.5 cm) lengths. Set aside.
* ❖ In saucepan over medium-high heat, bring 1-1/2 cups (375 mL) water to boil.
* ❖ Add asparagus; cover and cook until tender, about 4 minutes.
* ❖ Reserving cooking liquid, drain asparagus; set aside.
* ❖ Add enough water to cooking liquid to make 1-1/2 cups (375 mL).
* ❖ In same pan, bring stock, saffron (if using), and cooking liquid just to simmer over medium heat; reduce heat to low and keep warm.

- ❖ In separate large, shallow saucepan, melt 1 tbsp (15 mL) of the butter over medium heat; cook onion, carrot, zucchini, salt and pepper until vegetables are tender, about 4 minutes.
- ❖ Add rice, stirring to coat grains.
- ❖ Add wine; cook, stirring constantly, until all liquid is absorbed.
- ❖ Add stock mixture, 1/2 cup (125 mL) at a time, stirring after each addition until all liquid is absorbed and rice is creamy and tender, 20 minutes.
- ❖ Stir in remaining butter; add peas, Parmesan cheese, parsley and reserved asparagus.
- ❖ Cook, stirring, until risotto is creamy but still fluid and vegetables are hot, about 2 minutes.

64.   PEPPER CORN PAELLA

This vegetarian main dish makes a terrific meal with crusty rolls and a crunchy-crisp marinated salad. Prep time for this dish is about 15 minutes and cook time about 45 minutes for a total of about 1 hour yielding you about 4 servings.

Ingredients:

1 tbsp (15 mL) olive oil
1 onion, chopped
2 garlic cloves, minced
1 cup (250 mL) short grain rice
1/4 tsp (1 mL) turmeric
2 cups (500 mL) warm vegetable stock
1/4 tsp (1 mL) each sea salt and pepper
1 sweet green pepper
1 sweet red pepper
2 plum tomatoes
1-1/2 cups (375 mL) corn kernels
chopped fresh parsley

✳ How to prepare:

* ❖ In large nonstick skillet or paella pan, heat oil over medium heat; cook onion, garlic, rice and turmeric for 4 minutes or until onion is softened.
* ❖ Stir in stock, salt and pepper; bring to boil.
* ❖ Reduce heat, cover and simmer for 10 minutes.
* ❖ Meanwhile, cut green and red peppers in half lengthwise; remove core and membranes.
* ❖ Cut in half crosswise; cut lengthwise into strips.
* ❖ Core and chop tomatoes.
* ❖ Stir peppers and tomatoes into pan; cook, covered, for 15 minutes or until rice is almost tender.
* ❖ Stir in corn; cook, covered for about 5 minutes or until liquid has evaporated.
* ❖ Garnish with parsley.

65.   CHICK-PEA BURGERS

A tasty alternative to a meat burger, you'll love this grain and-legume burger. I'm always looking for creative ways to avoid red meat and I am a huge burger lover. This recipe will take you 20 minutes of prep time and about 15 minutes of cooking time for a total of 35 minutes yielding you 6 burgers.

Ingredients:

1 can (19 oz/540 mL) chickpeas, drained
1 cup (250 mL) cooked rice
1/3 cup (75 mL) grated onion
1/3 cup (75 mL) grated carrot
1/3 cup (75 mL) grated zucchini
1/4 cup (60 mL) dry breadcrumbs
1 egg, beaten
1 clove garlic, minced
2 tbsp (30 mL) tahini or peanut butter
1 tbsp (15 mL) lemon juice
1/2 tsp (2 mL) sea salt
1/4 tsp (1 mL) pepper
1/4 tsp (1 mL) dry mustard
3 whole wheat pita breads

✱ How to prepare:

- ❖ In large bowl and using potato masher, mash chickpeas coarsely; stir in rice, onion, carrot, zucchini, bread crumbs, egg, garlic, tahini, lemon juice, sea salt, pepper and mustard.
- ❖ Shape into six 3/4-inch (2 cm) thick patties.
- ❖ Place on greased grill over medium-high heat; cook for about 5 minutes per side or until golden brown.
- ❖ Halve pita breads; place burger in each pocket.

66. EGG SALAD SANDWICHES

This egg salad sandwich recipe is tops for being low in fat. Made with celery, light mayo and sour cream this makes a great lunch for work. Prep time is about 10 minutes and cook time is about 35 minutes for a total of 45 minutes and will provide you with 6 sandwiches.

Ingredients:

6 eggs
1/4 cup (60 mL) chopped celery
2 tbsp (30 mL) minced green onion
4 tsp (18 mL) light mayonnaise
4 tsp (18 mL) light sour cream
1 tbsp (15 mL) minced fresh parsley
1/4 tsp (1 mL) turmeric
1/4 tsp (1 mL) sea salt
1 Pinch cayenne pepper
6 slices whole wheat bread

✻ How to prepare:

- ❖ In saucepan, cover eggs with water; bring to boil.
- ❖ Remove from heat, cover and let stand for 20 minutes.
- ❖ Drain and chill under cold running water.
- ❖ Shell eggs; separate 3 yolks from whites and reserve for another use.
- ❖ Finely chop remaining eggs and whites.
- ❖ In bowl, combine chopped eggs, celery, green onion, mayonnaise, sour cream, parsley, turmeric, salt and cayenne.
- ❖ Spread on bread.

67.   VEGETARIAN HUMMUS BURGERS

Another meatless burger that you will enjoy, prep time takes about 20 minutes and cooking time will take about 30 minutes for a total of 50 minutes but will yield you 4 burgers.

Ingredients:

1/2 cup (125 mL) bulgur
1 can (19 oz /540 ml) chickpeas, drained and rinsed
2 tbsp (30 mL) lemon juice
1 clove garlic, minced
1/2 tsp (2 mL) sea salt
1/2 tsp (2 mL) ground cumin
1/4 tsp (1 mL) ground coriander
1/4 tsp (1 mL) ground pepper
1 egg
1/2 cup (125 mL) chopped roasted or fresh sweet red peppers
1/4 cup (60 mL) dry bread crumbs
2 tbsp (30 mL) chopped fresh parsley
1 tbsp (15 mL) olive oil
4 crusty buns whole wheat

✲ How to prepare:

- ❖ Pour 1 cup (250 mL) boiling water over bulgur; cover and let stand for 10 minutes. Drain well.
- ❖ In food processor, finely chop chickpeas.
- ❖ Add bulgur, lemon juice, garlic, salt, cumin, coriander, pepper and egg; pulse to combine.
- ❖ Stir in red pepper, bread crumbs and parsley.
- ❖ Shape into 8 patties.
- ❖ In nonstick skillet, heat half of the oil over medium-high heat; cook patties, in batches and adding remaining oil, for 4 to 6 minutes per side or until golden.

- ❖ For the tahini: Mix 1/4 cup (50 mL) each water and tahini (sesame paste), 1 tsp (5 mL) grated lemon rind, 2 tbsp (25 mL) lemon juice, 1 tsp (5 mL) chopped fresh parsley, 1 clove garlic, minced, and pinch sugar (optional).
- ❖ Stir in up to 2 tbsp (25 mL) more water if desired. Makes 1/2 cup (125 mL)

68. GRILLED VEGETABLE SUBMARINES

A quick tasty sub you can take to work for your lunch, prep time is about 15 minutes and cook time is about 5-10 minutes depending how you like to grill your vegetables for a total time of about 25 minutes which will yield you 4 subs.

Ingredients:

2 zucchinis
1 eggplant
1/2 sweet onion
1 sweet red pepper
1 sweet yellow pepper
3 tbsp (45 mL) extra virgin olive oil
2 tbsp (30 mL) minced fresh basil
1/2 tsp (2 mL)sea salt
1/2 tsp (2 mL) pepper
1/4 cup (60 mL) light mayonnaise
1 minced clove of garlic
4 submarine sandwich buns, preferably whole wheat if you can find
4 romaine leaves

✳ How to prepare:

- ❖ Cut zucchini lengthwise into 1/4-inch (5 mm) thick slices; place in large bowl.
- ❖ Cut eggplant and onion crosswise into 1/4-inch (5 mm) thick slices; add to bowl.
- ❖ Core, seed and cut red and yellow peppers into eighths; add to bowl.
- ❖ Add oil, 1 tbsp (15 mL) of the basil, salt and pepper; toss to coat.
- ❖ Place vegetables on greased grill over medium-high heat or 6 inches (15 cm) from broiler; close lid and grill or broil, turning once, until tender, about 5 minutes.
- ❖ Meanwhile, in small bowl, whisk together mayonnaise, garlic and remaining basil.
- ❖ Cut buns in half lengthwise; spread cut sides with mayonnaise mixture.
- ❖ Layer lettuce and grilled vegetables on bottom halves; sandwich with tops.
- ❖ You can add sliced provolone cheese or goat cheese. You can also grill the sandwiches. Just omit lettuce and grill until cheese is melted, about 3 minutes per side.

69.   LEMONY QUINOA SALAD

One of my favorite salads, this baby will take you 20 minutes of prep time and about 10 minutes of cooking time for a total of 30 minutes and yielding you 6 servings. Lime juice and cilantro give a refreshing kick, while quinoa and black beans provide tasty vegan protein.

Ingredients:

1 cup quinoa
2 cups water
1/4 cup extra-virgin olive oil
2 limes, juiced
2 teaspoons ground cumin
1 teaspoon sea salt
1/2 teaspoon red pepper flakes, or more to taste
1 1/2 cups halved cherry tomatoes
1 (15 ounce) can black beans, drained and rinsed
5 green onions, finely chopped
1/4 cup chopped fresh cilantro
sea salt and ground black pepper to taste

✳ How to prepare:

- ❖ Bring quinoa and water to a boil in a saucepan.
- ❖ Reduce heat to medium-low, cover, and simmer until quinoa is tender and water has been absorbed, 10 to 15 minutes.
- ❖ Set aside to cool.
- ❖ Whisk olive oil, lime juice, cumin, 1 teaspoon salt, and red pepper flakes together in a bowl.
- ❖ Combine quinoa, tomatoes, black beans, and green onions together in a bowl.
- ❖ Pour dressing over quinoa mixture; toss to coat.
- ❖ Stir in cilantro; season with salt and black pepper.
- ❖ Serve immediately or chill in refrigerator.

70.   GRILLED VEGETABLE QUINOA SALAD

Another tasty variation which will take you about 15 minutes of prep time and about 40 minutes of cooking time for a total of about 55 minutes and will yield you about 4 to 6 servings to enjoy.

Ingredients:

1 cup (250 mL) quinoa
1 sweet red pepper, quartered
1 sweet yellow pepper, quartered
1 zucchini, cut lengthwise in 1/2-inch thick strips
12 asparagus spears, trimmed
1/2 cup (125 mL) Light feta cheese, crumbled
1/4 cup (60 mL) toasted pumpkin seeds
3 tbsp (45 mL) chopped fresh cilantro

Chipotle Vinaigrette:
Chipotle Vinaigrette:

3 tbsp (45 mL) olive oil
2 tbsp (30 mL) red wine vinegar
1 canned chipotle pepper in adobo sauce, minced
2 tsp (10 mL) liquid honey
1/2 tsp (2 mL) ground cumin
1/4 tsp (1 mL) sea salt
1/4 tsp (1 mL) pepper

✳ How to prepare:

- ❖ Soak quinoa in cold water for 3 minutes; drain in sieve.
- ❖ In saucepan, bring 1-1/2 cups salted water to boil; stir in quinoa and return to boil.
- ❖ Reduce heat to low; cover and simmer until no liquid remains, 12 to 15 minutes.
- ❖ Remove from heat and fluff with fork; cover and let stand for 5 minutes.

- ❖ Spread on small tray and let cool for 10 minutes.
- ❖ Chipotle Vinaigrette: Meanwhile, whisk together oil, vinegar, chipotle pepper in adobo sauce, honey, cumin, salt and pepper. Set aside.
- ❖ In large bowl, toss together red and yellow peppers, zucchini, asparagus and 3 tbsp of the vinaigrette until coated.
- ❖ Place on greased grill over medium heat; close lid and grill until charred and tender, 4 to 6 minutes for asparagus, 10 to 12 minutes for peppers and zucchini.
- ❖ Cut into large chunks and return to bowl.
- ❖ Add remaining dressing, quinoa, half of the feta cheese, the pumpkin seeds and cilantro; stir until incorporated.
- ❖ Sprinkle with remaining feta.
- ❖ Serve immediately.

71. BROCCOLI AND CHEESE CASSEROLE

A nice casserole for a pot-luck or as a holiday side dish, simple and delicious, takes you about prep time of 15 minutes and 45 minutes of cooking time for a total of 1 hour yielding you about 4 to 6 portions.

Ingredients:

2 bunches broccoli, cut into florets
4 tablespoons of butter
3 ½ tablespoons of whole wheat flour
1 cup of milk
1 cup extra sharp cheese, shredded
½ cup bread crumbs
Olive oil for drizzling
Sea salt and pepper to taste

✶ How to prepare:

- ❖ Preheat oven to 350°
- ❖ Parboil broccoli: Chop broccoli into small pieces.
- ❖ Put into boiling water and let cook for 1-2 minutes only (take out when they are bright green!)
- ❖ Drain and rinse in really cold water until they are cool so they don't continue to cook.
- ❖ In a saucepan on low heat, melt butter, add the flour and stir until a consistent texture.
- ❖ It should start to smell slightly nutty.
- ❖ Slowly pour in the milk and stir.
- ❖ Season with sea salt and pepper.
- ❖ Fold in the sharp cheese and allow to get all melty and delicious.
- ❖ In small bowl, toss bread crumbs in a drizzling of olive oil.
- ❖ Lightly grease a casserole dish, layer your broccoli evenly, pour the cheesy sauce over top then sprinkle with breadcrumbs.
- ❖ Bake for 30 minutes or until the breadcrumbs are golden brown and cheese starts to bubble.

72.   VEGETARIAN PESTO PIZZA

This vegetarian pesto pizza recipe uses pesto instead of tomato sauce, and is topped with feta, artichokes and kalamata olives for a Mediterranean and Greek inspired fusion vegetarian pizza! Yum! Prep time is about 10 minutes and cooking time is about 15 minutes for a total of 25 minutes yielding you an entire pizza.

Ingredients:

1 15 - inch pre-made pizza crust
1/2 cup vegetarian pesto sauce
6 ounce feta cheese, crumbled
1 6 ounce jar artichokes, drained and chopped
1/3 cup hydrated sun-dried tomatoes, sliced
1/2 cup chopped kalamata olives

✻ How to prepare:

- ❖ Pre-heat oven to 400 degrees.
- ❖ Spread pesto sauce over crust.
- ❖ Sprinkle on feta cheese.
- ❖ Add artichokes, sun-dried tomatoes and olives.
- ❖ Bake for 15 minutes or until heated through.

73.   FRENCH BREAD VEGETABLE PIZZA

Everyone loves pizza, and piling your pizza high with vegetables means you can enjoy a healthy pizza anytime. Using French bread instead of a pizza crust, you can get this healthy vegetarian pizza recipe in the oven quickly. Prep time is about 10 minutes and cooking time about 10 minutes for a total of 20 minutes of your time, providing you with an entire pizza to divide anyway you like.

Ingredients:

1 one pound loaf French bread
1 cup pizza sauce
1 to 2 cups shredded mozzarella cheese
1 4 ounce can sliced mushrooms, drained
1 16 ounce can artichoke hearts, drained
1/2 large green pepper, sliced
1/2 large red or yellow pepper, sliced
1/2 cup chopped red onion
1 2 ounce can sliced black olives, drained
black pepper to taste

✶ How to prepare:

- ❖ Pre-heat oven to 350 degrees.
- ❖ Slice loaf in half, length-wise, and spread each half with equal amounts of ingredients.
- ❖ Sprinkle lightly with black pepper.
- ❖ Bake for 7 to 10 minutes, or until cheese melts.
- ❖ Slice each half into fourths.

74. GRATED MOZZARELLA VEGETARIAN PIZZA

I'm a big pizza fan, cause it tastes so good and it's easy to make. Prep time for this baby is only 15 minutes and cook time is about 12 minutes for a total of just 27 minutes of your time. This recipe will yield you an entire pizza whereby you can slice as many portions as you desire.

Ingredients:

1 pizza crust
1 cup (250 mL) pizza sauce
½ cup (125 mL) marinated artichoke hearts, cut in quarters
½ cup (125 mL) sliced mushrooms
¼ cup (60 mL) sliced onion
10 black olives, pitted and sliced
Pinch of oregano
1 ½ cups (375 mL) shreddedCanadian Mozzarella
½ green bell pepper, sliced
1 large tomato, thinly sliced

✳ How to prepare:

- ❖ Preheat oven to 450 °F (230 °C).
- ❖ Place crust on a lightly oiled pizza pan, pizza stone or cookie sheet.
- ❖ Cover with sauce.
- ❖ Add artichoke hearts, mushrooms, onion and olives.
- ❖ Season with oregano.
- ❖ Cover with Canadian Mozzarella.
- ❖ Top with pepper and tomato slices.
- ❖ Bake for 10 to 12 minutes.

75. CHEDDAR & ONION GRILLED CHEESE

With caramelized onions, aged cheddar cheese and apple slices, the humble grilled cheese sandwich is transformed into gourmet fare! Prep time for this recipe is about 10 minutes and cook time about 15 minutes for a grand total of 25 minutes yielding you 4 sandwiches to enjoy for either lunch or when you are on the go!

Ingredients:

8 slices bread, preferably whole wheat toast bread
4 tbsp. butter
About 1/2 cup to 3/4 cup caramelized onions
4 thick slices aged cheddar cheese
2 apples, thinly sliced
4 handfuls baby arugula
3 tbsp. olive oil
1 1/2 tbsp. balsamic vinegar
Sea salt and freshly ground pepper, to taste

✳ How to prepare:

- ❖ Assemble 4 sandwiches with caramelized onion, cheese and apple slices.
- ❖ Butter the outer sides of the bread slices.
- ❖ Heat a large frying pan over medium heat.
- ❖ Add sandwiches (in batches if needed) and cook until bread is golden brown and cheese melts, about 3 to 4 minutes per side.
- ❖ If needed, finish sandwiches in a preheated 350 degree F. oven to melt the cheese.
- ❖ To make a quick arugula salad: Drizzle arugula with olive oil and balsamic vinegar. Season with salt and pepper and toss to combine.
- ❖ Serve grilled cheese sandwiches with arugula salad or your favorite Soup.
- ❖ For the caramelized onions: Heat 1/4 cup olive oil in a large heavy-bottomed pan over medium to medium low heat. Add 5 thinly sliced onions. Cook onions, stirring regularly, until dark golden brown and caramelized, about 1 hour.

76. TOFU BURGER

Low calorie burger that only takes 20 minutes of prep time and 10 minutes of cooking time for a total of 30 minutes yielding you about 8 burger patties.

Ingredients:

2 eggs
32 oz firm tofu
2 stalks celery (minced)
1 minced onion
1 tbsp chili powder
1 tbsp ground cumin
1 tbsp red curry paste
1 tbsp minced garlic
2 cups rolled oats
1 tbsp olive oil

✳ How to prepare:

❖ Beat the eggs in a mixing bowl until smooth.
❖ Mix in the tofu, celery, onion, chili powder, cumin, curry paste, garlic, and oats with your hands until the tofu has broken into fine pieces, and the mixture is evenly blended. Form into 8 patties.
❖ Heat the vegetable oil in a large, nonstick skillet over medium heat.
❖ Cook the patties until crispy and golden brown on each side, about 5 minutes per side.

77. SUPER-STAR VEGGIE BURGER

You are gonna love this burger, takes about 20 minutes of prep time and 10 minutes of cooking time for a grand total of only 30 minutes of your precious time. This recipe will yield you 8 burgers to enjoy!

Ingredients:

15 1/2 oz garbanzo beans (drained and mashed)
8 fresh basil leaves (chopped)
1/4 cup oat bran
1/4 cup quick cooking oats
1 cup brown rice (cooked)
14 oz firm tofu
5 tbsps barbeque sauce
1/2 tsp sea salt
1/2 tsp black pepper (ground)
3/4 tsp garlic powder
3/4 tsp sage (dried)
2 tsps olive oil

✻ How to prepare:

- ❖ In a large bowl, stir together the mashed garbanzo beans and basil.
- ❖ Mix in the oat bran, quick oats, and rice; the mixture should seem a little dry.
- ❖ In a separate bowl, mash the tofu with your hands, trying to squeeze out as much of the water as possible.
- ❖ Drain of the water, and repeat the process until there is hardly any water worth pouring off.
- ❖ It is not necessary to remove all of the water.
- ❖ Pour the barbecue sauce over the tofu, and stir to coat.
- ❖ Stir the tofu into the garbanzo beans and oats.
- ❖ Season with salt, pepper, garlic powder, and sage; mix until well blended.

- ❖ Heat the oil in a large skillet over medium-high heat.

* Form patties out of the bean mixture, and fry them in hot oil for about 5 minutes per side.
* Serve as you would burgers.

78.   LENTIL SOUP

One of my favorite soups in the world, nothing beats my grand-mother's recipe, I try to have this soup for supper once a week with some whole wheat pita bread and a small piece of feta cheese. Prep time for this recipe is about 15 minutes and cooking time about 45 minutes for a grand total of 1 hour of your time which will provide you with 6 servings.

Ingredients:

1 tablespoon olive oil
1 medium celery stalk, small dice
1 medium carrot, peeled and small dice
1/2 medium yellow onion, small dice
3 medium garlic cloves, minced
Sea salt
Freshly ground black pepper
1 quart low-sodium vegetable broth
1 (15-ounce) can diced tomatoes with their juices
1 1/4 cups lentils (any color except red), rinsed
1 bay leaf
1/4 teaspoon finely chopped fresh thyme leaves
1 teaspoon red wine vinegar
2 ounces spinach leaves (about 1/2 a bunch)

✳ How to prepare:

* ❖ Heat the oil in a large saucepan over medium heat until shimmering, about 3 minutes.
* ❖ Add the celery, carrot, and onion and cook, stirring occasionally, until the vegetables have softened, about 10 minutes.
* ❖ Stir in the garlic and cook until fragrant, about 1 minute.
* ❖ Season with several generous pinches of sea salt and pepper.
* ❖ Add the broth, tomatoes with their juices, lentils, bay leaf, and thyme and stir to combine.

- ❖ Cover and bring to a simmer, about 15 minutes.
- ❖ Once simmering, reduce the heat to low and continue simmering, covered, until the lentils and vegetables are soft, about 15 minutes more.
- ❖ Taste and season with more salt or pepper as needed, then stir in the vinegar.
- ❖ Add the spinach and stir until wilted.
- ❖ If you prefer a creamier texture, purée half of the soup in a blender and add it back to the pot.

79. BASMATI RICE

Quick rice recipe for either a quick lunch or can be served as a side dish, basmati rice is my personal favorite rice by the way, prep time takes about 20 minutes and cooking time about another 20 minutes for a total of 40 minutes of your time, yielding you about 4 servings.

Ingredients:

1 3/4 cups water
1 cup basmati rice
1/4 cup frozen green peas
1 teaspoon cumin seeds

✱ How to prepare:

- In a saucepan bring water to a boil.
- Add rice and stir.
- Reduce heat, cover and simmer for 20 minutes.
- When rice is cooked, stir in peas and cumin.
- Cover and let stand for 5 minutes.

80. INDIAN-STYLE BASMATI RICE

I'm a big fan on Indian and this is a great recipe that can be had alone or as a side-dish, of course butter chicken comes to mind. Prep time for this recipe is 10 minutes and cook time is 25 minutes for a total time of 35 minutes of your time, yielding you about 6 servings.

Ingredients:

1 1/2 cups basmati rice
2 tablespoons olive oil
1 (2 inch) piece cinnamon stick
2 pods green cardamom
2 whole cloves
1 tablespoon cumin seed
1 teaspoon sea salt
2 1/2 cups water
1 small onion, thinly sliced

✳ How to prepare:

* ❖ Place rice into a bowl with enough water to cover.
* ❖ Set aside to soak for 20 minutes.
* ❖ Heat the oil in a large pot or saucepan over medium heat.
* ❖ Add the cinnamon stick, cardamom pods, cloves, and cumin seed.
* ❖ Cook and stir for about a minute, then add the onion to the pot.
* ❖ Saute the onion until a rich golden brown, about 10 minutes.
* ❖ Drain the water from the rice, and stir into the pot.
* ❖ Cook and stir the rice for a few minutes, until lightly toasted.
* ❖ Add sea salt and water to the pot, and bring to a boil.
* ❖ Cover, and reduce heat to low.
* ❖ Simmer for about 15 minutes, or until all of the water has been absorbed.
* ❖ Let stand for 5 minutes, then fluff with a fork before serving.

81. MUSHROOM LENTIL BARLEY STEW

The flavors blend nicely to give it a wholesome earthy flavor that is unbelievably vegetarian. Prep time for this recipe is 15 minutes and cook time about 12 hours for a grand total of 12 hours and 15 minutes of your time. This recipe will yield you about 8 servings.

Ingredients:

2 quarts vegetable broth
2 cups sliced fresh button mushrooms
1 ounce dried shiitake mushrooms, torn into pieces
3/4 cup uncooked pearl barley
3/4 cup dry lentils
1/4 cup dried onion flakes
2 teaspoons minced garlic
2 teaspoons dried summer savory
3 bay leaves
1 teaspoon dried basil
2 teaspoons ground black pepper
sea salt to taste

✳ How to prepare:

- ❖ In a slow cooker, mix the broth, button mushrooms, shiitake mushrooms, barley, lentils, onion flakes, garlic, savory, bay leaves, basil, pepper, and sea salt.
- ❖ Cover, and cook 4 to 6 hours on High or 10 to 12 hours on Low.
- ❖ Remove bay leaves before serving.

82.   INDIAN CURRIED BARLEY PILAF

This is a delicious and savory curried barley dish that I hope you enjoy. Prep time is only 5 minutes while cooking time is about 50 minutes for a total of 55 minutes of your time. The recipe will yield you about 6 servings.

Ingredients:

1/4 cup butter
1 onion, diced
1 1/2 cups pearl barley
1/2 teaspoon ground allspice
1/2 teaspoon ground turmeric
1/4 teaspoon curry powder
1/2 teaspoon sea salt
1/8 teaspoon ground black pepper
3 1/2 cups chicken broth
1/4 cup slivered almonds
1/4 cup raisins (optional)

✳ How to prepare:

- ❖ Melt butter in a large skillet placed over medium-high heat.
- ❖ Add the onion and barley; cook, stirring frequently, until the onion begins to soften, about 5 minutes.
- ❖ Stir in the allspice, turmeric, curry powder, sea salt, and black pepper.
- ❖ Pour in the chicken broth, and bring to a simmer.
- ❖ Cover skillet with lid, and reduce heat to low; simmer until the barley is tender, about 30 to 40 minutes.
- ❖ Fluff the pilaf with a fork, and gently stir in the slivered almonds and raisins.

83.   BULGUR WHEAT WITH DRIED CRANBERRIES

Very simple yet tasty side that goes well with grilled or roasted chicken or you can even have it stand alone. Any type of dried fruit can be used in place of the dried cranberries. Prep time for this recipe is 10 minutes and cooking time about 15 minutes for a total of 25 minutes while providing you with 2 servings.

Ingredients:

1 cup water
1/2 cup dry bulgur wheat
1 1/2 tablespoons chicken bouillon granules
1 teaspoon butter
1/4 cup dried cranberries

* How to prepare:

* Bring water to a boil in a pot, and mix in bulgur, bouillon granules, and butter.
* Cover pot, reduce heat to low, and simmer 15 minutes.
* Fluff cooked bulgur with a fork, and gently mix in the dried cranberries.

84.   VEGETABLE BULGUR SALAD

A very popular Turkish/Middle Eastern salad that is good for you and you shall enjoy. Prep time is 15 minutes and cook time is about 5 minutes for total time of 20 minutes yielding you about 6 servings.

Ingredients:

1 cup fine bulgur
1 cup boiling water
2 tablespoons olive oil
1 onion, finely chopped
2 large tomatoes, finely chopped
1 cucumber, diced
2 green bell peppers, finely chopped
1 red bell pepper, finely chopped
7 green onions, finely chopped
1/2 cup minced fresh parsley
1/2 cup minced fresh mint leaves
1 teaspoon red pepper flakes, or to taste
juice of 1 fresh lemon
2 tablespoons pomegranate molasses

✴ How to prepare:

- ❖ Place the bulgur in a bowl; stir in the boiling water.
- ❖ Cover and let stand for 20 minutes.
- ❖ Meanwhile, heat 2 tablespoons olive oil in a skillet over medium heat.
- ❖ Stir in the chopped onion; cook and stir until the onion has softened and turned translucent, about 5 minutes.
- ❖ Drain the bulgur and return it to the bowl.
- ❖ Add the cooked onion, chopped tomatoes, cucumber, green and red bell peppers, green onions, parsley, mint, and red pepper flakes.

- ❖ Drizzle with 2 tablespoons olive oil, the lemon juice, and the pomegranate molasses.
- ❖ Toss gently until the salad is thoroughly combined.
- ❖ Serve immediately, or refrigerate until serving.

85. GREEN BEANS WITH LEMON AND GARLIC

This simple recipe takes only 5 minutes of prep time and about 12 minutes of cooking time for a total of 17 minutes of your time and will yield you 6 servings. Green beans are very filling, so you will get your protein and many other nutrients too!

Ingredients:

2 pounds green beans
1 tablespoon extra-virgin olive oil
3 tablespoons butter
2 large garlic cloves, minced
1 teaspoon red pepper flakes
1 tablespoon lemon zest
Sea salt and freshly ground black pepper

✳ How to prepare:

❖ Blanch green beans in a large stock pot of well salted boiling water until bright green in color and tender crisp, roughly 2 minutes.
❖ Drain and shock in a bowl of ice water to stop from cooking.
❖ Heat a large heavy skillet over medium heat.
❖ Add the oil and the butter.
❖ Add the garlic and red pepper flakes and saute until fragrant, about 30 seconds.
❖ Add the beans and continue to saute until coated in the butter and heated through, about 5 minutes.
❖ Add lemon zest and season with sea salt and pepper.

86. GREEN BEANS AND POTATOES IN CHUNKY TOMATO SAUCE

One of my favorite dishes from my childhood and a popular greek home recipe. Prep time is only 10 minutes and cooking time about 15 minutes for a total of 25 minutes of your time and providing you with about 8 servings.

Ingredients:

1 1/2 tablespoons olive oil
1 garlic clove, minced
1 1/2 cups diced red potato
1/2 cup chopped celery
1/2 teaspoon sea salt
1 1/4 pounds green beans, trimmed
1/4 cup water
1/3 cup chopped fresh cilantro
3/4 pound plum tomatoes, peeled and coarsely chopped
1/4 teaspoon freshly ground black pepper
1/4 teaspoon ground red pepper

✱ How to prepare:

- ❖ To peel tomatoes, score the skin by making a small X on the bottom side with a sharp knife.
- ❖ Place tomato in boiling water for 30 seconds.
- ❖ Remove tomato using a slotted spoon; immediately submerge in a bowl of ice water.
- ❖ Let stand for one minute.
- ❖ Heat olive oil in a large skillet over medium-high heat.
- ❖ Add garlic to pan; sauté 30 seconds, stirring constantly.
- ❖ Add potato, celery, sea salt, and beans; sauté 1 minute.
- ❖ Add 1/4 cup water; cover and cook 5 minutes or until beans are crisp-tender.
- ❖ Add cilantro and tomatoes.

❖ Cover, reduce heat, and cook 4 minutes or until tomatoes begin to soften, stirring occasionally.
❖ Stir in peppers.

87.   MANDARIN ORANGE AND ALMOND DELIGHT

Great tasting salad that will take you 15 minutes of prep time and about 5 minutes of cooking time for a total of 20 minutes.

Ingredients:

1/2 cup blanched slivered almonds
1 (11 ounce) can mandarin oranges, juice reserved
2 tablespoons olive oil
2 tablespoons apple cider vinegar
12 ounces mixed salad greens

✳ How to prepare:

- ❖ Heat a skillet over medium-high heat.
- ❖ Add almonds, and cook, stirring frequently, until lightly toasted.
- ❖ Remove from heat, and set aside.
- ❖ In a small bowl, whisk together 2 tablespoons reserved mandarin orange juice, oil, and vinegar.
- ❖ In a large salad bowl, toss together the toasted almonds, mandarin oranges and mixed salad greens.
- ❖ Season with some sea salt

88. APPLE ALMOND CRUNCH SALAD

This easy-to-assemble salad combines the great crunch of apples and almonds with the sweetness of golden raisins and the unique texture of feta cheese. Prep time for this salad is just 10 minutes and there is no cooking time involved, so 10 minutes total yielding you about 6 servings.

Ingredients:

1 (10 ounce) package mixed salad greens
1/2 cup slivered almonds
1/2 cup crumbled feta cheese
1 cup tart apple, cored and chopped
1/4 cup sliced red onion
1/4 cup golden raisins
2 tbsp of olive oil
2 tbsp of apple cider vinegar

✳ How to prepare:

❖ In a large salad bowl, combine the salad greens, almonds, feta cheese, apple, red onion and raisins.
❖ Toss to blend.
❖ Apply salad dressing of olive oil and apple cider vinegar to individual servings.

89.   CALIFORNIA CHERRY AND WALNUT SALAD

A simple light and sweet salad with goat cheese, dried cherries and walnuts. Prep time takes 10 minutes and there is no cooking time, this recipe will yield you about 4 salads.

Ingredients:

1 (10 ounce) bag mixed salad greens
2 tbsp olive oil
2 tbsp apple cider vinegar
1/4 cup walnut pieces
2 tablespoons dried tart cherries
4 ounces goat cheese, sliced
1/4 pound cooked chicken breast strips (optional)

✳ How to prepare:

- ❖ Toss the salad greens, walnut pieces, and dried cherries together in a large bowl.
- ❖ Add the olive oil and apple cider vinegar
- ❖ Divide the salad into individual salad bowls or plates.
- ❖ Garnish each salad with two slices of goat cheese and a few strips of chicken breast.

90. AVOCADO EGG SALAD

A fun and filling salad that will take you about 20 minutes of prep time and no cooking time which will yield you approximately 12 servings.

Ingredients:

6 avocados - peeled, pitted, and cubed
1 teaspoon fresh lemon juice
5 hard-cooked eggs, chopped
1/2 red onion, minced
1/2 cup light mayonnaise
1 tablespoon milk
3 hard-cooked eggs, sliced
1/2 teaspoon paprika

✳ How to prepare:

❖ Toss avocado cubes with lemon juice in a serving bowl; mix avocado with chopped egg and onion.
❖ Whisk together the mayonnaise and milk; add to avocado mixture and gently mix.
❖ Arrange the remaining eggs sliced atop the salad in rows.
❖ Sprinkle top with paprika.

91. EGG SALAD WITH GREEN PEAS

This is a good and fulfilling egg dish that is best served warm. Prep time is only 15 minutes while cooking time is 30 minutes for a grand total of 45 minutes of your time. This recipe will yield you 4 servings.

Ingredients:

9 eggs
1 cup frozen green peas, thawed
3/4 cup diced celery
2 tablespoons chopped pimento
2 tablespoons chopped onion
1 1/2 cups dry bread crumbs
1 cup mayonnaise
1/3 cup milk
1/2 teaspoon garlic salt
salt and pepper to taste
2 tablespoons butter

✱ How to prepare:

- ❖ Preheat oven to 400 degrees F (200 degrees C).
- ❖ Place eggs in a saucepan and cover with cold water.
- ❖ Bring water to a boil; cover, remove from heat, and let eggs stand in hot water for 10 to 12 minutes.
- ❖ Remove from hot water, cool, peel and chop.
- ❖ In a large bowl, combine the eggs, peas, celery, pimento, onion, 1 cup bread crumbs, mayonnaise, milk, garlic salt, salt and pepper.
- ❖ Mix well and pour into a 1 quart casserole dish.
- ❖ Melt butter and fry remaining 1/2 cup bread crumbs until lightly browned.
- ❖ Sprinkle over casserole and bake at 400 degrees F (200 degrees C) for 30 minutes.

92. MIXED BEAN SALAD

This bean salad is really filling and you definitely get your dose of protein for the day with it. Prep time is only 30 minutes and cook time clocks in a 5 minutes for a total of 35 minutes of your time. This salad will yield you about 10 servings.

Ingredients:

1 (14.5 ounce) can green beans, drained
1 (14.5 ounce) can wax beans, drained
1 (15.25 ounce) can red kidney beans, drained
1 (15 ounce) can garbanzo beans, drained
1 (15 ounce) can black beans, drained
1 red onion, chopped
1 green bell pepper, chopped
3/4 cup apple cider vinegar
3/4 cup olive oil
3/4 teaspoon ground dry mustard
1/2 teaspoon dried tarragon
1 1/2 teaspoons dried cilantro

✱ How to prepare:

- ❖ In a large bowl, layer the beans, onion and green pepper. Set aside.
- ❖ In a small saucepan, mix the vinegar, olive oil, mustard, tarragon and cilantro.
- ❖ Cook and stir over medium heat.
- ❖ Remove from heat and pour over bean mixture.
- ❖ Stir until all ingredients are coated.
- ❖ This is best if it is left to marinate for a few hours in the refrigerator, and stirred occasionally.

93.   RED BEAN SALAD WITH FETA AND PEPPERS

A tasty, nutrient-packed salad that can be eaten by itself or as a side dish. Makes a great lunch the next day too! Prep time takes about 20 minutes and there is no cooking time involved. This recipe will yield you about 4 servings.

Ingredients:

1 (15 ounce) can kidney beans
1 red bell pepper, chopped
2 cups chopped cabbage
2 green onions
1 cup crumbled feta cheese
1/3 cup chopped fresh parsley
1 clove garlic, minced
2 tablespoons lemon juice
1 tablespoon olive oil

✳ How to prepare:

- ❖ Rinse kidney beans under cold water. Drain well.
- ❖ In a large salad bowl, combine beans, red pepper, cabbage, onions, feta, parsley, garlic, lemon juice, and olive oil.

94.   PASTA CHICKPEA SALAD

Simple and tasty salad that packs protein so you don't get hungry after an hour. Prep time is 15 minutes while cooking time is 35 minutes for a grand total of 50 minutes. This recipe will yield you about 6 portions.

Ingredients:

1 (16 ounce) package rotelle whole wheat pasta

2 tablespoons extra virgin olive oil

1/2 cup chopped oil-cured olives

2 tablespoons minced fresh oregano

2 tablespoons chopped fresh parsley

1 bunch green onions, chopped

1 (15 ounce) can garbanzo beans (chickpeas), drained and rinsed

1/4 cup apple cider vinegar

1/2 cup grated Parmesan cheese

sea salt and pepper to taste

✳ How to prepare:

- ❖ Bring a large pot of salted water to a boil, add pasta and cook until al dente.
- ❖ Drain and rinse under cold water. Set aside to chill.
- ❖ In a large skillet heat the olive oil over medium low heat.
- ❖ Add the olives, oregano, parsley, scallions and chickpeas.
- ❖ Cook over low for about 20 minutes. Set aside to cool.
- ❖ In a large bowl toss the pasta with the chickpea mixture.
- ❖ Add the vinegar, grated cheese and sea salt and pepper to taste.
- ❖ Let sit in refrigerator overnight.
- ❖ When ready to serve taste for seasoning and add more vinegar, olive oil and salt and pepper if desired.

95.   GREEK SALAD

This is an incredibly good Greek salad recipe, nice and tangy and even better in the summer when you use fresh vegetables! Prep time is 20 minutes and there is no cooking involved. This recipe will provide you with about 6 servings.

Ingredients:

1 head romaine lettuce- rinsed, dried and chopped
1 red onion, thinly sliced
1 (6 ounce) can pitted black olives
1 green bell pepper, chopped
1 red bell pepper, chopped
2 large tomatoes, chopped
1 cucumber, sliced
1 cup crumbled feta cheese
6 tablespoons olive oil
1 teaspoon dried oregano
1 lemon, juiced
ground black pepper to taste

✶ How to prepare:

- ❖ In a large salad bowl, combine the Romaine, onion, olives, bell peppers, tomatoes, cucumber and cheese.
- ❖ Whisk together the olive oil, oregano, lemon juice and black pepper.
- ❖ Pour dressing over salad, toss and serve.

96.   CUCUMBER-WATERMELON SALAD

This cool, refreshing summer salad is so delicious! Sweet and tangy at the same time, you can even add a piece of feta cheese in it if you like, very popular salad in Greece. Prep time is 15 minutes and cooking time is another 15 minutes for a total of 30 minutes of your time. This recipe makes 10 servings.

Ingredients:

6 cups cubed seeded watermelon
4 cups cubed English cucumber
1 teaspoon sea salt
1 tablespoon white sugar(optional)
1/2 cup balsamic vinegar

✸ How to prepare:

❖ Place the watermelon and cucumber cubes in a large bowl, and gently toss with the salt and sugar.
❖ Drizzle with balsamic vinegar and toss to coat.
❖ Refrigerate for 15 minutes, then gently toss one last time before serving.
❖ Add feta cheese (optional)

97.   KALE, QUINOA, AND AVOCADO SALAD

Steaming the kale removes some of the bitterness. A quartet of super foods (kale, quinoa, avocado, and olive oil) make this a healthy meal. Prep time is 25 minutes and cook time is about 15 minutes for a total of 40 minutes to prepare this salad. This recipe will yield you about one large salad.

Ingredients:

2/3 cup quinoa
1 1/3 cups water
1 bunch kale, torn into bite-sized pieces
1/2 avocado - peeled, pitted, and diced
1/2 cup chopped cucumber
1/3 cup chopped red bell pepper
2 tablespoons chopped red onion
1 tablespoon crumbled feta cheese
Dressing
1/4 cup olive oil
2 tablespoons lemon juice
1 1/2 tablespoons Dijon mustard
3/4 teaspoon sea salt
1/4 teaspoon ground black pepper

✳ How to prepare:

- ❖ Bring the quinoa and 1 1/3 cup water to a boil in a saucepan.
- ❖ Reduce heat to medium-low, cover, and simmer until the quinoa is tender, and the water has been absorbed, about 15 to 20 minutes. Set aside to cool.
- ❖ Place kale in a steamer basket over 1 inch of boiling water in a saucepan.
- ❖ Cover saucepan with a lid and steam kale until hot, about 45 seconds; transfer to a large plate.
- ❖ Top kale with quinoa, avocado, cucumber, bell pepper, red onion, and feta cheese.
- ❖ Whisk olive oil, lemon juice, Dijon mustard, sea salt, and black pepper together in a bowl until the oil emulsifies into the dressing; pour over the salad.

98. BLACK BEAN SALAD

Love this salad which is very hearty since it packs the protein and carbs evenly for a power lunch! Prep time is 30 minutes and cook time is another 30 minutes for a total of 1 hour. This recipe will yield you 6 servings.

Ingredients:

2/3 cup uncooked basmati rice
1/3 cups water
3/4 cup black beans, drained and rinsed
1 large tomato, seeded and diced
3/4 cup shredded Cheddar cheese
1/3 cup sliced green onions
1/3 cup olive oil
1/4 cup apple cider vinegar
1 tablespoon diced jalapeno peppers
1/2 teaspoon white sugar
sea salt to taste
1 avocado - peeled, pitted and diced

✳ How to prepare:

- ❖ In a saucepan, bring water to a boil. Add rice and stir.
- ❖ Reduce heat, cover and simmer for 20 minutes.
- ❖ Remove from heat and chill.
- ❖ In a large bowl, mix together the rice, beans, tomato, cheese and green onion.
- ❖ In a small bowl, whisk together the olive oil, vinegar, peppers, sugar and sea salt.
- ❖ Pour over the rice mixture and toss to coat.
- ❖ Cover and refrigerate salad for 30 minutes.
- ❖ Top with avocado just before serving.

99. SOME GOUT SMOOTHIES THAT LOWER URIC ACID

Just use the following ingredients and juice them in the blender of your choice and enjoy a healthy gout friendly smoothie or juice.

1-Ingredients:

1 medium-sized cucumber
2 ribs of celery
a slice of lemon
1 inch of fresh ginger root

2-Ingredients:

1 carrot
2 green apples
2 celery sticks
½ cucumber
¼ lemon
½ inch of ginger root

3-Ingredients: (Raw Cherry Smoothie)

300 grams cherries
2 bananas
1 cup of water or coconut water

4-Ingredients:

½ cucumber
¼ cup of whole cranberries

1 cup cherries

1 cup watermelon

½ cup of alfalfa sprouts

1 cup blueberries